International Series on Public Policy

Series Editors
Guy Peters
Department of Political Science
University of Pittsburgh
Pittsburgh, PA, USA

Philippe Zittoun
Research Professor of Political Science
LET-ENTPE, University of Lyon
Lyon, France

The International Series on Public Policy—the official series of International Public Policy Association, which organizes the International Conference on Public Policy—identifies major contributions to the field of public policy, dealing with analytical and substantive policy and governance issues across a variety of academic disciplines. A comparative and interdisciplinary venture, it examines questions of policy process and analysis, policymaking and implementation, policy instruments, policy change and reforms, politics and policy, encompassing a range of approaches, theoretical, methodological, and/or empirical. Relevant across the various fields of political science, sociology, anthropology, geography, history, and economics, this cutting edge series welcomes contributions from academics from across disciplines and career stages, and constitutes a unique resource for public policy scholars and those teaching public policy worldwide.

More information about this series at
http://www.palgrave.com/gp/series/15096

Justin Parkhurst • Stefanie Ettelt
Benjamin Hawkins
Editors

Evidence Use in Health Policy Making

An International Public Policy Perspective

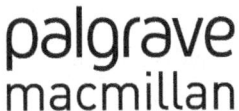

Editors
Justin Parkhurst
London School of Economics
and Political Science
London, UK

Stefanie Ettelt
London School of Hygiene
and Tropical Medicine
London, UK

Benjamin Hawkins
London School of Hygiene
and Tropical Medicine
London, UK

International Series on Public Policy
ISBN 978-3-030-06667-3   ISBN 978-3-319-93467-9 (eBook)
https://doi.org/10.1007/978-3-319-93467-9

© The Editor(s) (if applicable) and The Author(s) 2018. This book is published open access.
Softcover re-print of the Hardcover 1st edition 2018
Open Access This book is licensed under the terms of the Creative Commons Attribution 4.0 International License (http://creativecommons.org/licenses/by/4.0/), which permits use, sharing, adaptation, distribution and reproduction in any medium or format, as long as you give appropriate credit to the original author(s) and the source, provide a link to the Creative Commons license and indicate if changes were made.
The images or other third party material in this book are included in the book's Creative Commons license, unless indicated otherwise in a credit line to the material. If material is not included in the book's Creative Commons license and your intended use is not permitted by statutory regulation or exceeds the permitted use, you will need to obtain permission directly from the copyright holder.
The use of general descriptive names, registered names, trademarks, service marks, etc. in this publication does not imply, even in the absence of a specific statement, that such names are exempt from the relevant protective laws and regulations and therefore free for general use.
The publisher, the authors and the editors are safe to assume that the advice and information in this book are believed to be true and accurate at the date of publication. Neither the publisher nor the authors or the editors give a warranty, express or implied, with respect to the material contained herein or for any errors or omissions that may have been made. The publisher remains neutral with regard to jurisdictional claims in published maps and institutional affiliations.

This Palgrave Macmillan imprint is published by the registered company Springer Nature Switzerland AG
The registered company address is: Gewerbestrasse 11, 6330 Cham, Switzerland

Preface

There have been many calls for better evidence and better use of evidence in health policy making in specific countries and internationally. Much attention has been paid to the variable quality of policy-relevant research, the claims to validity of different research designs, and the independence and conflicts of interest of researchers (Cartwright and Hardie 2012; Evans 2003; Marmot 2004; Petticrew and Roberts 2003). However, differences in the availability of independent, high quality, research only provides one of several possible answers to the complex problem of explaining why some policies in particular contexts, and at certain points in time, appear to be more aligned with evidence from research than others.

It is an empirical observation that the idea and rhetoric of 'evidence-based', or 'evidence-informed' policymaking are more prevalent in some countries and in some policy fields than others. In Britain, for example, evidence-informed policy became an official government aspiration since the 1999 White Paper "Modernising Government" (HM Government 1999), while in Germany official discourse is largely unaffected by explicit appeals to evidence per se; although in practice there are many examples in which experts, expertise and research contribute to policy decisions. The health sector particularly embraces the language of evidence use, given its successful history of shaping clinical practice through the embrace of the methods of 'evidence based medicine' (Klein 2000; Berridge and Stanton 1999) – and the experience of the medical field has led to calls for other sectors to emulate its methods and approach to evidence use (HM Government 2013). Indeed, global health advocacy is often built around scientific expertise and evidence in the form of research findings, which play a crucial role in informing decisions of international organisations such as the World Health Organization (Oxman et al. 2007; D'Souza and Newman 2012). Similarly, international donor agencies often utilise the rhetoric of evidence use to justify their aid expenditures or policy choices in the health sector, often presenting the image of a comprehensively rational ideal by which health policy decisions can or should be made.

Yet at national level, the picture is often vastly different, with local practices, partisan interests and national politics seen to stand in the way of better uses of evidence. In this respect, the health sector may appear no different from other policy fields, despite the idea that health policy decisions can use evidence to guide choices the same way that clinical practice has done through the methods of evidence based medicine. This raises important questions such as: Why are some countries more likely than others to take account of findings from research in the development of health policy? Why are some more successful than others in creating, and institutionally embedding, an architecture that supports long-term evidence use and a wider norm of evidence informed policy making? Does it matter whether governments have more or less executive power, compared to parliaments and the judiciary, to oversee and shape policy decisions? And how do we explain these differences and analyse the 'bigger picture' of evidence use in national policy and politics?

For many advocating for 'evidence-based policymaking' today, politics is conceptualised as something detrimental to evidence use. From this perspective, political concerns, priorities and timetables, along with party political interests, are hurdles that derail efforts of making policy more evidence informed or even more 'rational'. However, there is often little clarity as to what is meant by 'politics' in those authors who simplify the concept as a 'barrier' to evidence use.

Increasingly, however, a number of authors investigating the relationship between evidence and policy have concluded that we need to engage with the nature of the policy process more fully and, in particular, the political nature of the policy making process (Ettelt and Mays 2011; Oliver et al. 2014; Strassheim and Kettunen 2014; Cairney 2016; Parkhurst 2017). Often starting from a policy studies or public policy perspective, these works argue that to see politics as a simple 'barrier' to evidence use presents a false dichotomy between political and rational-technocratic forms of decisions making. It is also to engage in a form of wishful thinking that we can somehow step outside of 'politics' to arrive at optimal, evidence-led policy decisions. Politics is not the barrier to identifying the correct policy path to follow (a path presumably indicated by the evidence), but the process through which societies identify and agree upon which path to take in the first place. It is a process through which policy objectives, solutions to problems and resource allocation are debated, considered, agreed, or disputed. Instead of a barrier to evidence use, politics must be accepted as a necessary and inevitable condition of the policy making domain. Political contestation over values, ideas and political priorities thus characterise all forms of policy decision. This is particularly so in the context of squeezed public finances and limited time in which not all demands can be met and choices must be made, between often highly worthy claims to public resources.

It is therefore of critical importance to health sector actors to realise that health policy decisions are not placed outside political systems, but rather made within existing political systems and institutional settings. In this volume we argue that it is equally critical to consider the nature of political systems influencing the use of, and opportunities for, evidence to inform health policy decisions. A public policy lens thus not only requires recognition of the multiplicity of social concerns at stake within a health policy decision, it also mandates consideration of the structures, rules, processes and norms, i.e. the political institutions, in place in different country settings to understand when, why, and how pieces of evidence may be used to inform health decisions.

The book is based on a five-year research project supported by the European Research Council entitled 'Getting Research into Policy in Health' (the GRIP-Health project) which aimed to improve the understanding and practices of evidence use by examining health policy processes in six different countries. These countries were selected to allow for a number of comparisons both in relation to different regime types, different levels of socio-economic development and different approaches to health policy-making. The book investigates how governments in these countries used evidence to inform policy decisions, the type of contestation policy-makers are exposed to, and the scope of actors that have an influence on health policy-making in various institutional forms, both within and beyond government. By examining evidence use in different country contexts we can better understand the institutional factors and settings that shape policy processes and therefore shape the opportunities for building and embedding mechanisms that institutionalise the use of evidence in policy processes.

It is in the nature of these types of research endeavours to start with a broad perspective which then becomes more focused on individual case study analyses. This book attempts to combine both perspectives: The first part brings together a number of in-depths analyses of health policy decisions in individual countries, using a spread of health policy topics to explore the institutional dynamics in high-income countries (Germany, England), middle-income countries (Ghana, Colombia) and lower-income countries (Ethiopia, Cambodia[1]).

The second part provides an overview of the dynamics within relevant institutional settings such as the structures in which evidence use is embedded in Ministries of Health, the role of parliaments and the judiciaries as key institutions of the (democratic) state in relation to evidence use, and the power divergence associated with aid dependency in low income countries and its potential impact on research uptake in policy decisions.

Chapters share a public policy perspective that is concerned with the political nature of contested decisions and/or the institutional structures in which decisions are made. Cases in each chapter apply these ideas to analyse or reflect on evidence use for health decision making in each setting. The directions each case study or country analysis takes, however, is unique and a reflection of the realities of the nature of the problems and issues emerging in each situation. Ultimately, then, the book applies a multidisciplinary lens to institutional analysis of the role of evidence in health policy, which we hope our readers will find interesting and illuminating.

London, UK

Stefanie Ettelt
Benjamin Hawkins
Justin Parkhurst

References

Berridge, V., and J. Stanton. 1999. Science and policy: Historical insights. *Social Science & Medicine* 49: 1133–1138.

Cairney, P. 2016. *The politics of evidence-based policy making*. London: Palgrave Macmillan.

---

[1] At the time of the research programme's initiation, Cambodia was classified as a low income country according to the World Bank, but subsequently its national income rose to current classification as lower-middle income.

Cartwright, N., and J. Hardie. 2012. Evidence-based policy: Doing it better. A practical guide to predicting if a policy will work for you. Oxford, UK: Oxford University Press.
D'Souza, B., and R.D. Newman. 2012. Strengthening the policy setting process for global malaria control and elimination. *Malaria Journal* 11: 1–3.
Ettelt, S., and N. Mays. 2011. Health services research in Europe and its use for informing policy. *Journal of Health Services Research and Policy* 16: 28–60.
Evans, D. 2003. Hierarchy of evidence: A framework for ranking evidence evaluating healthcare interventions. *Journal of clinical nursing* 12: 77–84.
HM Government. 1999. *Modernising government*. London: The Stationery Office.
HM Government. 2013. *What works: Evidence centres for social policy*. London: Cabinet Office.
Klein, R. 2000. From evidence-based medicine to evidence-based policy? *Journal of Health Services Research & Policy* 5: 65.
Marmot, M.G. 2004. Evidence based policy or policy based evidence? Willingness to take action influences the view of the evidence – Look at alcohol. *BMJ* 328: 906–907.
Oliver, K., T. Lorenc, and S. Innvær. 2014. New directions in evidence-based policy research: A critical analysis of the literature. *Health Research Policy and Systems* 12: 34.
Oxman, A.D., J.N. Lavis, and A. Fretheim. 2007. Use of evidence in WHO recommendations. *The Lancet* 369: 1883–1889.
Parkhurst, J. 2017. *The politics of evidence: From evidence-based policy to the good governance of evidence*. Abingdon: Routledge.
Petticrew, M., and H. Roberts. 2003. Evidence, hierarchies, and typologies: Horses for courses. *Journal of Epidemiology and Community Health* 57: 527–529.
Strassheim, H., and P. Kettunen. 2014. When does evidence-based policy turn into policy-based evidence? Configurations, contexts and mechanisms. *Evidence & Policy: A Journal of Research, Debate and Practice* 10: 259–277.

ACKNOWLEDGEMENTS

This work is part of the Getting Research Into Policy in Health (GRIP-Health) project, supported by a grant from the European Research Council (Project ID#282118).

Contents

1 Studying Evidence Use for Health Policymaking
  from a Policy Perspective   1
  Justin Parkhurst, Stefanie Ettelt, and Benjamin Hawkins

2 The Many Meanings of Evidence: A Comparative Analysis
  of the Forms and Roles of Evidence Within Three Health
  Policy Processes in Cambodia   21
  Helen Walls, Marco Liverani, Kannarath Chheng, and Justin
  Parkhurst

3 The Role of Evidence in Nutrition Policymaking
  in Ethiopia: Institutional Structures and Issue Framing   51
  Helen Walls, Deborah Johnston, Elisa Vecchione, Abdulfatah
  Adam, and Justin Parkhurst

4 The Use of Evidence in Health Policy in Ghana:
  Implications for Accountability and Democratic
  Governance   75
  Elisa Vecchione and Justin Parkhurst

5 Using Evidence in a Highly Fragmented Legislature:
  The Case of Colombia's Health System Reform   91
  Arturo Alvarez-Rosete and Benjamin Hawkins

6 The Politics of Evidence Use in Health Policy Making in Germany: The Case of Regulating Hospital Minimum Volumes 111
Stefanie Ettelt

7 Electronic Cigarettes Regulation in the UK: A Case Study in Evidence Informed Policy Making 137
Benjamin Hawkins

8 Ministries of Health and the Stewardship of Health Evidence 155
Justin Parkhurst, Arturo Alvarez-Rosete, Stefanie Ettelt, Benjamin Hawkins, Marco Liverani, Elisa Vecchione, and Helen Walls

9 Evidence Use and the Institutions of the State: The Role of Parliament and the Judiciary 185
Stefanie Ettelt

10 Evidence and Policy in Aid-Dependent Settings 201
Justin Parkhurst, Siobhan Leir, Helen Walls, Elisa Vecchione, and Marco Liverani

11 Conclusion: Reflecting on Studying Evidence Use from a Public Policy Perspective 221
Justin Parkhurst, Benjamin Hawkins, and Stefanie Ettelt

Index 239

CHAPTER 1

Studying Evidence Use for Health Policymaking from a Policy Perspective

Justin Parkhurst, Stefanie Ettelt, and Benjamin Hawkins

INTRODUCTION

Individuals working within the health sector very often see their work as guided by collectively shared normative values. In particular there is an overarching goal of improving people's health. Indeed the field of public health has been defined as "the science and art of preventing disease, prolonging life and promoting health through organized efforts of society" (Acheson 1988, p. 1). This is often linked, either implicitly or explicitly, to a concern for improving health equity (or reducing health inequalities) – for instance within the World Health Organization's calls to achieve 'health for all' (Detels and Tan 2015; Whitehead 1991). In recent decades, efforts to improve population health and to reduce health inequalities within countries and globally between states, have been linked with calls for evidence based policy (EBP). Drawing on the idea of evidence based

J. Parkhurst (✉)
London School of Economics and Political Science, London, UK
e-mail: j.parkhurst@lse.ac.uk

S. Ettelt • B. Hawkins
London School of Hygiene and Tropical Medicine, London, UK
e-mail: stefanie.ettelt@lshtm.ac.uk; ben.hawkins@lshtm.ac.uk

© The Author(s) 2018
J. Parkhurst et al. (eds.), *Evidence Use in Health Policy Making*,
International Series on Public Policy,
https://doi.org/10.1007/978-3-319-93467-9_1

medicine (EBM), health policy actors see engagement with policy-relevant evidence to identify more effective, and by extension cost effective, interventions as the way to achieve their overarching policy objectives.

EBM as a concept is based on the idea that medicine should be practiced by making "conscientious, explicit, and judicious use of current best evidence in making decisions about the care of individual patients" (Sackett et al. 1996, p. 71). The origin of this idea is often attributed to Archie Cochrane, who wrote in the early 1970s about the need to use evidence of effectiveness to guide clinical practice (Cochrane 1972), although it was in 1993 that the formal establishment of the Cochrane Collaboration further served to provide both a global repository of evidence for specific clinical interventions, and an authority for best practices on how to review or select evidence to inform medical practice (Starr et al. 2009).

The notion of 'conscientious, explicit, and judicious' evidence use is relevant to consider in this context. From the earliest origins of the EBM movement, there was recognition that it is not necessarily appropriate to rely solely on research evidence when making decisions on diagnoses and medical treatment. Professional experience and judgement on the part of medical practitioners, in light of the evidence base and relevant inferences from this, remain important (Sackett et al. 1996). However, over time, the principles of EBM have gravitated towards specific types of evidence with clear preferences for certain study designs – encapsulated in so-called 'hierarchies of evidence' (Petticrew and Roberts 2003) – reflecting concerns about the internal validity of studies and the potential for biased outcomes that, in medicine, "routinely lead to false positive conclusions about efficacy" (Sackett et al. 1996, p. 72).

The EBM movement has, overall, been heralded as a triumph and is credited with ensuring that medical treatments produce beneficial results, particularly compared to the past, when many interventions were promoted solely on the basis of hypotheses of potential cause and effect that may, in fact, have been incorrect (Howick 2011). The Academy of Medical Royal Colleges, for instance, has argued that EBM "is the key to the success of modern Healthcare" (Sense About Science and Academy of Royal Medical Colleges 2013, p. 1), co-authoring a report providing examples of how EBM has improved health outcomes on a range of issues from HIV/AIDS treatment to emergency allergy care and mental health treatment (Sense About Science and Academy of Royal Medical Colleges 2013).

The success of EBM has been seen by many authors as the inspiration for calls to expand the concept to other forms of decision making including 'evidence based policymaking' in health and other social policy areas

(Berridge and Stanton 1999; Wright et al. 2007; Lin and Gibson 2003; Parkhurst 2017). This is despite recognition of the challenges in appropriating ideas from clinical practice and applying them to shape policymaking processes. For example, Black (2001) urged the medical community to 'proceed with care' with the idea of evidence based policy due to the qualitatively different nature of policymaking compared to medicine. A number of other authors have similarly argued that the political realities of policy decisions mean policy cannot simply be 'based' on evidence in the same way as clinical decisions and that the notion of a linear-rational relationship between evidence and policy is a fallacy (c.f. Lewis 2003; Hammersley 2005; Greenhalgh and Russell 2009).

Russell et al. (2008), for example, have explained that:

> ...academic debate on health care policy-making continues to be couched in the dominant discourse of evidence-based medicine, whose underlying assumptions – that policies are driven by facts rather than values and these can be clearly separated; that 'evidence' is context-free, can be objectively weighed up and placed unproblematically in a 'hierarchy'; and that policymaking is essentially an exercise in decision science. (p. 40)

These messages appear to have had only limited impact on the conceptual vocabulary of health policy making and scholarship. Despite these warnings, the language of 'evidence based policymaking' has become firmly established in health policy discourses, particularly in the United Kingdom (UK), Canada, and within many global health networks. As such, recent publications have continued to critique examples of the oversimplified or idealised embrace of evidence on which to 'base' policy (c.f. Hammersley 2013; Cartwright and Hardie 2012; Parkhurst 2017). In addition, recent systematic reviews have found limited engagement with the political nature of policymaking to help explain evidence use. Oliver, Innvaer, and Lorenc (2014a) concluded from one such review that while studies of evidence use have spread from health to other sectors, few works actually engage with aspects of the policy process or provide sufficient details to draw firm conclusions. In a related paper, the authors argue that:

> The agenda of 'getting evidence into policy' has side-lined the empirical description and analysis of how research and policy actually interact in vivo. Rather than asking how research evidence can be made more influential, academics should aim to understand what influences and constitutes policy, and produce more critically and theoretically informed studies of decision-making. (Oliver et al. 2014b, p. 1)

Another review by Liverani et al. (2013) (undertaken as part of the research programme making up this volume), similarly reviewed literature on evidence use related to health policymaking and found few examples that explicitly addressed politics to help explain the use of evidence to inform health policymaking.

Given this state of affairs, this book aims to contribute to a greater understanding of the political nature of policymaking and how it shapes the potential for, and resultant outcomes of, evidence use in health policymaking. In particular, we focus on scientific evidence arising from research and related systematic processes of data collection (e.g. data collection for monitoring the health system) as our principle subject. This is because, while we recognise that the term 'evidence' can take many meanings – including personal experience and legal argumentation – it is the formal results of research activity and the application of the scientific method that have been seen as essential to the aspirations of both the EBM and the EBP movements.

We argue that while policy advocates have pursued their normative goals of improving health outcomes through 'better' policymaking, associated with reliance on research evidence, this has brought about a discourse that too narrowly focuses on certain conceptions of what counts as policy-relevant evidence. In addition, it overstates the role which evidence is able to play in the policy making process whilst paying insufficient attention to the politics of that process, including the competition of values, ideologies, and policy objectives which cannot themselves be determined by recourse to evidence.

There is thus a need to examine the complex interrelationship of evidence use and politics to form a more nuanced conception of the health policy process. This starts from an explicit recognition of the fundamentally political nature of the policy process that recognises that, while evidence can and should be an important factor informing policy debates, it cannot provide the sole basis for policy decisions or is usually insufficiently suited to resolve policy conflicts.

The Multiple Meanings of 'Use' of Research Evidence

The point of departure for developing our conceptualisation of how evidence informs policy is to start by questioning what it means to 'use' evidence in policymaking. Unlike clinical decision making, which often involves a choice between clearly circumscribed interventions for a fairly specific purpose (to improve patient outcomes), using evidence to inform policy usually does not fit this model. More often than not, policy is not a clearly delineated object, and there may be disagreement not just about the preferred policy 'solution', but also about the nature and definition of the problem to be addressed.

That evidence use in policymaking is not entirely compatible with notions of instrumental rationality has been known for some time. Indeed, Carol Weiss (1979) described a number of different meanings of research utilisation in the late 1970s. She discusses social science research more widely, but her models of research use are conducive to health policy research as well. In particular, she identifies seven variants of research utilisation, including a 'knowledge-driven' model in which basic research identifies new social problems; a 'political' model in which research is strategically used to achieve pre-existing goals; and an 'enlightenment' model in which research influences broader thinking more generally.

The model that perhaps best aligns with the current dominant rhetoric in the health sector, however, is Weiss' so-called 'problem solving' model of research utilisation, which sees direct application of a study's findings (for example findings from an evaluation of an intervention) to inform a specific policy decision (for example, a decision about which intervention to fund). Weiss, however, notes that it requires a tremendous, and incredibly rare, alignment of circumstances to see research used in this way. Indeed, this requires the identification, and agreement on the definition of a problem that policy and research are expected to address. In practice, of course, both problems and their solutions tend to be highly contested. For example, to some, health inequalities run counter to accepted norms of social justice and are thus identified as legitimate targets of government intervention, while for others inequalities are seen as the outcome of personal choices and thus beyond the remit of the state. Similarly, for some, governments are seen to have a responsibility to care for all, while for others government intervention in health is seen as an unwelcome overreach or intrusion on individual and market freedoms.

Contestation between groups who have different sets of values or beliefs in many ways is at the heart of many theories of policy change which perceive policymaking as a competitive process rather than a technocratic one (Sabatier 2007; John 1998). Yet it has been argued that the level and nature of these competitive environments can incentivise the manipulation of scientific or empirical evidence to achieve desired political goals (Parkhurst 2016). As a result, strategic, rather than instrumental uses of evidence appear commonplace in many policy arenas where political interests exist – often decried as 'policy-based evidence-making' and seen as a fundamental challenge to the ideal rational use of evidence that many social sector stakeholders champion (Marmot 2004; Strassheim and Kettunen 2014).

Nutley et al. (2007) have also provided a comprehensive mapping of many potential meanings of evidence use/utilisation that includes, but expands on Weiss' original concepts. They identify that "the most common image of research use is of an instrumental process that involves the direct application of research to policy and practice decisions" (p. 34). However, the authors detail a number of other ways to conceptualise research use beyond this simple view. This includes producing typologies of evidence use (similar to Weiss' (1979) model), as well as models which see practices of evidence use as a continuum from more conceptual to more instrumental uses, or instead considering evidence use as a process or series of stages rather than as one or more types.

These works highlight the limitations of instrumental approaches to evidence use, even if this continues to be held up as an ideal in many academic and professional circles. Yet mapping the different ways research and evidence are used does not, on its own, explains neither why we see different forms of evidence use arise at different times and in different contexts, nor what constitutes a 'good use of evidence' in particular policy areas. This is particularly important when reflecting on the specific goals of health sector actors, and the common belief across that sector about how robust use of evidence (and in particular of research evidence) will help to achieve those goals. In this volume we thus attempt to move forward from these initial mapping exercises to directly engage with the political nature of policymaking to reflect on how evidence is used within the health sector. This approach allows explicit consideration of the systems in place that work to provide evidence to policy decision makers, or seek to improve evidence use in some way.

A Public Policy Perspective

A public policy perspective on evidence use accepts that political dimensions of health policymaking will affect the relevance and use of evidence within those policy processes. Yet the policy sciences are a broad field, consisting of a wide range of theories and concepts that can each be used to provide insights into policy processes and outcomes. Thus calling for more public policy insights requires consideration of how precisely to apply this field of work to study evidence use in a comparative perspective.

Previous authors have engaged with theories of policy change to help explain when or how evidence might be used within policy processes. Yet what is apparent from these works is that there is a tremendous range of theories that could provide insights in one or another way to this question. Cairney (2016) highlights the relevance of a number of theories, frameworks, and approaches including: multiple streams theory, punctuated equilibrium theory, social constructionism, narrative frameworks, the advocacy coalitions framework, studies of policy transfer or diffusion, and complexity theory (see Cairney 2016, chapter 2). Cairney, however, embraces the usefulness of the concept of bounded rationality in particular, due to his work having a central focus on policy makers' perspectives and a need to overcome the comprehensive rationality underlying the evidence-based policymaking thinking. Smith (2013a) reviews many of the same theories as Cairney, including theories of policy change, but focuses on the 'power of ideas' to shape what is considered relevant evidence, and to affect the roles and actions of policy actors for two contrasting health policy issues: health inequalities and tobacco control.

The variety of policy studies theories thus provides a range of explanatory perspectives to consider different questions about policymaking and policy change. For example, if one was concerned with how evidence fits within ongoing processes of policy change, Kingdon's multiple streams approach or the Advocacy Coalitions Framework could be the most appropriate approaches to adopt. We are sympathetic to this wide variety of approaches and the insights they can provide into particular questions of evidence use.

However, in this volume we focus on two particular approaches derived from the policy sciences. First, we engage with the contested nature of policy decisions between multiple stakeholders who may be pursuing different interests, and conceptualising policy problems in different ways. Second we consider the influence of the political institutions that work to shape when and how particular forms of evidence influence policy decisions in different settings. Our decision to focus on these factors arose primarily from a desire to explore how the political nature of the policy process affects evidence use in different settings; as well as a desire to understand which forms of evidence use arise in different institutional contexts.

Politics as Power and Contestation

One of the most widespread criticisms of calls for 'evidence based policymaking' comes from authors who point to the inherently contested nature of policy decisions. Unlike in clinical decision situations, policy is, as Lasswell (1990 [1936]) classically observed, about 'who gets what, when and how', emphasising the possibility of conflict over the distributive effects of policy. Ultimately, policy-making is about power and influence, and the ability of policy actors to generate or withhold support and influence an outcome. It is therefore not possible to separate policymaking from politics. Scholars have historically noted that policymaking represents decisions, made on behalf of society, to decide on what collective goals that society should pursue (Brecht 1959). As such it can be argued that these processes require some form of democratic legitimation that would typically be derived from ensuring that multiple interests are articulated or considered in the decision making process (even if some are excluded in the final choice of outcome) (Young 2000). In such a process, however, competing stakeholders participating in this process will seek to frame the terms of policy debates in way amenable to the objectives in order to shape decisions (Russell et al. 2008), with the recourse to 'evidence' serving as one mechanism through which policy discourses can be shaped in favour of (or against) a particular outcome.

In many instances there are wide asymmetries of power between different actors with obvious consequences for their ability to influence the definition of the policy problem, for example through issue framing, and the type of intervention put in place to address them (Lukes 2005). Transnational corporations, for example the global tobacco and alcohol industries, have enjoyed high degrees of success in shaping policy and the wider debates which surround policy decisions, not simply through direct lobbying, but through their use of media consultants, public relations and corporate social responsibility campaigns (Hawkins and Holden 2013).

The importance of issue framing in policy debates is thus critical to understand, both in relation to the construction of policy-relevant conceptualisations of evidence and in relation to what can be achieved by appeals to evidence in the context of highly contested policy debates. The framing of an issue can shape the way in which a policy problem is seen; the very essence of what it 'is' for the observer. This affects what the correct and legitimate policy response to this is considered to be, and thus what is identified as the most relevant body of evidence in assessing the policy problem under consideration and the proposed responses (c.f. Bacchi 2009; Fischer 2003). If we accept multiple, often mutually exclusive, framings of policy problems are possible, each claiming support from different (sometime overlapping) bodies of evidence, then the impossibility of settling policy dilemmas through recourse to *the* evidence becomes acutely apparent. This is why Russell et al. (2008) noted that it is 'naively rational' to assume that evidence can simply direct policy making in a linear way, with Hammersley (2013) going so far as to claim that 'evidence-based policy' is nothing more than a slogan used to discredit opponents.

Recognising the contested nature of decision making means that the specific form of issue contestation, the strength of relevant interests, the power of stakeholders and their networks, and their ability to frame problems and solutions, can be expected to play important roles in shaping how evidence is used within health policymaking processes. From this perspective, the actors involved in policymaking take centre stage analytically, with regard to the interest they may represent, the strategies they pursue and the behaviours they display to achieve their desired outcome. Focusing on contestation therefore allows for a deeper analysis of the role of actors, their interests, and agency. It also allows an alternative conceptualization of evidence use in policy processes. As Weiss (1979, 1991) already observed, actors can use evidence strategically or tactically to support a decision and to delegitimise other positions that are not supported by evidence (or by evidence of the same methodological robustness). Likewise, it is conceivable that evidence is used to build support and generate 'buy-in' and consensus, especially from audiences that are likely to support the notion that evidence should be a key ingredient of policymaking. In practice such efforts can fail as well as succeed. It will therefore be difficult to clearly separate different uses of evidence, which may be simultaneously instrumental and strategic.

Lines of contestation can be studied through a variety of case study types, including analysis of a single health issue in a single context; of multiple health issues in a single context; or for the same health issue in different contexts. We have examples of all of these within this volume. However, policy contestation is merely a starting point to apply the policy sciences to the study of evidence use, even with the depth of conceptual insights this initial step allows. Our driving interest was not only to look at single decision events or policy choices, but to consider longer term and systemic uses of evidence within the health sector. This means recognition that evidence use in decision making is not just a single occurrence or event, but rather it is an ongoing process integral to the policy process. Thus the second main component to our conceptual approach is to engage with concepts of institutionalism in order to explore how institutions shape and direct the ongoing use of evidence affecting health decisions across multiple decision points and over longer time frames.

An Institutional Perspective to Analyse Evidence Use in Policy Processes

Lowndes and Roberts (2013) posit that "[i]nstitutions are central to the subject matter of political analysis (p. 1)," and, indeed, institutional analysis is well established in the fields of political analysis and international public policy comparisons, including comparisons of health systems and reforms (Immergut 1992; Tuohy 1999). Given its history with EBM, many look to the health sector in particular as leading other social sectors in its engagement with evidence use (Parkhurst 2017); but even in this field, only a small number of studies to date have directly analysed institutions in relation to evidence use for policy. Some of these have focussed on organisational arrangements that facilitate or hinder the uptake of pieces of evidence; for example in relation to drug policy in England and Scotland (Nutley et al. 2002), in health inequality policy in England (Smith 2013b), or, in relation to clinical practice, in routine nursing practice in US hospitals (Stetler et al. 2009). The interest in organisational arrangements is also reflected in some current work on organisational 'embeddedness' of evidence use as well within health policymaking bodies (c.f. Gonzales-Block 2013; Koon et al. 2013). Other work has looked at institutionalised processes of evidence use to inform fairly circumscribed sub-fields of health policy, such as coverage decisions relating to publicly funded health services and pharmaceuticals, with the use of health technology assessment (HTA) a prominent example (Garrido 2008; Turchetti et al. 2010).

However, our own systematic review of studies on evidence use, could find only a limited engagement with the concept of institutions, especially political institutions relevant to policymaking, to help explain the use of evidence in policymaking in the health-related literature (Liverani et al. 2013). This echoes an earlier finding by Nutley et al. (2002), who looked at public policy more broadly and concluded that "insufficient attention has been paid to the institutional arrangements for connecting research (and other evidence) to policy (p. 77)."

Therefore, we find that a significant gap in the literature still exists to consider institutions more directly in relation to their role in shaping evidence use for health policy making. In this volume, we draw on the broader concepts typical of new institutionalism, as explored by authors such as Peters (2005, 2008) and Lowndes and Roberts (2013), who see new institutionalism as a way to move beyond historical work that focussed solely on formal arrangements of political systems, to additionally consider how institutional rules, practices, and narratives work to shape policy actor behaviour.

From this perspective, and based on the analyses in the chapters that follow, we stipulate that institutional structures, norms, practices, and narratives will influence evidence use in policymaking in two ways. First, institutional arrangements will shape the processes of policymaking and thus determine which actors have access to policy and whose positions are considered relevant or legitimate. This can be formal, for example through stipulations as to who will be involved any given policy decision, or informal, with actors having an implicit understanding, or a shared perception, of the appropriateness of who should be involved in and who excluded from the decision process. This focus on the roles of key policy actors helps to capture the institutionalised features of policy contestation in different settings, akin to what Peters (2005) describes as a rational choice branch of new institutionalism which maintains a focus on policy actors pursuing their interests within institutional arrangements. We have used this perspective in a number of different countries to analyse how different institutional arrangements influence which stakeholders bring evidence of different kinds to policy processes, often in the pursuit of particular interests.

Second, efforts to improve the use of evidence in policymaking can themselves lead to the creation of new structures, rules, practices, and narratives that inform future policy decisions, i.e. evidence utilisation of one form or another can become institutionalised, described elsewhere as 'governing' how evidence is used (c.f. Hawkins and Parkhurst 2015; Parkhurst 2017). For example, governmental or non-governmental bodies have been set up in countries with the explicit aim of generating, assessing or synthesising evidence to develop a more consistent (and often a more instrumental) approach to evidence use in policy. In order to exercise their mandate, these bodies have, over time, created a set of rules and practices that guide how they execute their mandates and go about their tasks. These rules and practices are typically accompanied by ideas about the 'right' types of evidence (e.g. the 'hierarchy of evidence'), methods of appraisal and synthesis, and ways of using them in decision-making (c.f. Sutherland 2001; Petrisor and Bhandari 2007; Evans 2003; Borgerson 2009). Bodies such as these also operate with a legal framework set by government or legislatures, which can lead to instances where their decisions may be challenged or overridden by other political institutional structures (c.f. Chap. 5 in this volume and Ettelt forthcoming).

Critically exploring these concepts can utilise what Peters (2005) describes as normative institutionalism, which applies ideas such as March and Olsen's (1989, 2006) 'logics of appropriateness'. This concept is in many ways the antithesis of rational choice perspectives that see individuals as pursuing their own interests, and instead explores how, within institutional arrangements, individuals work towards outcomes guided by collective normative principles of what is seen to be the correct thing to do, or what is the right outcome to achieve. This can therefore be used to explore how practices play out within key administrative bodies in relation to dominant ideas about evidence use (or about evidence-based policymaking) within the health sector; and further allows consideration of how alternative logics play out when health related policymaking takes place across institutions and policy sectors with their own distinct normative goals.

Institutions can be formal and informal, as well as explicit and implicit, which means that at times they can be difficult to pin down analytically or observe empirically. Yet all permutations may play out in important ways to shape evidence use in different political contexts. Rules such as legislation would be at the formal, explicit end of the spectrum, while narratives and discourses about which behaviours of policy actors are appropriate are more likely to be informal (and potentially implicit). In combination, institutional elements form structures and logics that shape how actors behave, how they relate to each other, and how they relate to policy processes, both individually and collectively. Ultimately these factors can play important roles in shaping which of the many forms of evidence use arise in different health policy processes – be it instrumental uses in line with idealised views of the health community, strategic uses by policy actors to pursue their interests, or some other form or combination of the types of evidence use.

OUTLINE OF THE BOOK

The remainder of this book presents a set of chapters consisting of country case studies and comparative analyses that arose from a five-year research project supported by the European Research Council entitled 'Getting

Research into Policy in Health' (the GRIP-Health project). The project aimed to improve the understanding and practices of evidence use by examining health policy processes in six countries cutting across low, middle, and high income settings, as well as varying in their geographic location and administrative arrangements. Specifically cases come from Cambodia, Colombia, Ethiopia, Germany, Ghana, and the United Kingdom (analysed as the UK in Chap. 7, but more narrowly focussing on England in other comparative chapters).

The first set of chapters presents findings from individual country-focussed investigations. These examined one or more health policy topics, as well as processes of decision making, with explicit consideration of the contestation of the issues and/or the institutional arrangements in place that end up affecting the use of evidence.

Chapter 2 presents the first of our country examples with a case study from Cambodia that specifically looks at the differences in evidence use for three contrasting health policy issues – HIV/AIDS, tobacco control, and performance based financing of midwifery services. The chapter illustrates that despite the broad rhetorical embrace of the concept of evidence based policymaking within the health sector, the extent to which evidence is used in instrumental ways can vary substantially depending on the political realities of specific policy topics, including competing governmental interests in issues or the conceptual framing about what evidence is meant to achieve in different cases. The chapter considers the differing logics of actors in each policy process and how these shape evidence use for different health issues.

Chapter 3 follows with an analysis from Ethiopia that looks specifically at the challenges to multisectoral planning for nutrition in that country. It continues the concern over logics of appropriateness in relation to evidence use by reflecting on how different sectors (health, agriculture, finance, etc.) may see their goals and thus their perceptions of policy relevant evidence in different ways. The chapter also reflects on the constructed nature of the framing of nutrition policy in the country, which could reflect competing goals between differing policy sectors. Overall it considers how these features make multisectoral planning, and the use of evidence within such planning, a challenge.

Chapter 4 presents a case from Ghana that, rather than looking at a specific policy topic, focusses on a key part of the evidence advisory system of the country. Specifically, the Chapter investigates the institutional system in place which dictates how routine local data is used to inform annual health sector planning and policy reviews. The chapter considers how the data and evidence review process has been institutionalised in ways that not only shape which data and pieces of evidence inform certain planning activities, but which also may have governance implications in terms of the systems of accountability in the country, and the role or influence of international funding agencies.

In Chap. 5, a case study in Colombia further expands the institutional lens to look more broadly at the role of the legislature within ongoing health systems reform debates. The chapter also engages directly with the importance of policy contestation in shaping when evidence will, or will not, have a role in influencing legislative outcomes. The analysis illustrates that even though scientific evidence was found to be available to decision makers, it was unable to provide common ground or positions of compromise within the highly contested and fragmented health policy field.

Chapter 6 presents a case study from Germany that particularly explores the instrumental and strategic uses of evidence to inform debates about minimum service volumes in hospitals (i.e. whether facilities should have to provide a minimum number of procedures to be allowed to offer the service). The analysis illustrates how the interests of key actors can lead to strategic uses of evidence, but further highlights the dynamic relationship between evidence use and the political and institutional context, exploring how the legislative nature of policy-making, corporatism, and the role of the judiciary in Germany influence these uses of evidence in this case.

The final country case study in this section comes in Chap. 7 presenting the case of electronic cigarette policy in the UK. This case study focuses on the contested nature of policy debates, but further considers the importance of how alternative constructions or framings of the policy issue itself by competing groups may help to explain how evidence is used. The chapter then discusses why appeals to particular forms of evidence do not have the impact that many health actors might expect. It concludes by reiterating a core theme of this volume that the political nature of policy debates must be engaged with explicitly to understand evidence use for health policymaking.

Following these country specific chapters, we present a set of three comparative analyses that draw lessons from across multiple country cases to address key themes arising from the project. Chapter 8 begins with a direct consideration of the institutional systems in place that work to provide evidence to inform decision making by Ministries of Health. It begins by considering the roles that Ministries of Health have as stewards of national health care, considering how this can also extend to having a mandate to shape the evidence advisory systems which will inform health policy decisions. It then looks across all six of our country cases to consider whether such systems provide relevant information in a timely manner to key decision points. The chapter illustrates how key structural and practical differences exist between countries, and also notes that, at times, key health decisions lie outside the authority of Ministries of Health, providing further challenges to the roles that formalised evidence advisory systems might play to inform those decisions.

This recognition of non-ministerial authority over health decisions leads directly to Chap. 9, which discusses insights about the roles of legislatures and the judiciary in shaping evidence use for health decisions. The chapter draws out lessons from multiple country case studies to illustrate the different ways that these bodies may use evidence to classic ideas of instrumental or problem-solving use embraced by many health sector actors. Ultimately the chapter draws out just how different evidence use can look within national policy processes based on existing institutional systems embedded in the legal or constitutional frameworks of countries.

Chapter 10 presents the final comparative chapter, drawing lessons on evidence use in relation to the role and potential influence of international aid donors in our lower-income, aid-dependent case study countries (Ethiopia, Cambodia, and Ghana). The chapter draws out the importance of factors such as: the levels of local technical capacity, differing stakeholder framings of issues, and the influence of external actors on underlying systems of decision making. The chapter discusses how these were seen to affect which evidence was used and for what purposes – illustrating how the broader political economy of aid and development can play out in multiple ways in terms of evidence use in health policymaking.

Finally, Chap. 11 provides a discussion chapter that allows us to reflect on the issues raised in this introduction. We revisit what our cases show in terms of the many meanings of research utilisation, and consider what has been learned in terms of how political and institutional factors shape the form of evidence use arising in health policy processes. The chapter synthesises insights about how political contestation, issue construction, and institutional arrangements all work (and at times work together) to shape and direct evidence use. The chapter, however, concludes by recognising that the insights from this volume only present a starting point to understanding the politics of evidence use from a public policy perspective, merely scratching the surface of the many areas of research that can further be done in this field.

REFERENCES

Acheson, Donald. 1988. *Public health in England*. Report of the Committee of Inquiry into the future development of the public health function, The Stationary Office, London.
Bacchi, Carol Lee. 2009. *Analysing policy: What's the problem represented to be?* Frenchs Forest NSW: Pearson Australia.
Berridge, V., and J. Stanton. 1999. Science and policy: Historical insights. *Social Science & Medicine* 49 (9): 1133–1138.
Black, Nick. 2001. Evidence based policy: Proceed with care. *British Medical Journal* 323: 275–279.
Borgerson, Kirstin. 2009. Valuing evidence: Bias and the evidence hierarchy of evidence-based medicine. *Perspectives in Biology and Medicine* 52 (2): 218–233.
Brecht, Arnold. 1959. *Political theory: The foundations of twentieth-century political thought*. Princeton: Princeton University Press.
Cairney, Paul. 2016. *The politics of evidence-based policymaking*. London: Palgrave Pivot.
Cartwright, N., and J. Hardie. 2012. *Evidence-based policy: A practical guide to doing it better*. Oxford: Oxford University Press.
Cochrane, Archibald Leman. 1972. *Effectiveness and efficiency: Random reflections on health services*. Vol. 900574178. London: Nuffield Provincial Hospitals Trust.
Detels, Roger, and Chorh Chuan Tan. 2015. The scope and concerns of public health. In *The Oxford handbook of global public health*, ed. Roger Detels, Martin Gulliford, Quarraisha Abdool Karim, and Chorh Chuan Tan, 6th ed., 3–18. Oxford: Oxford University Press.
Ettelt S. forthcoming. Access to treatment and the constitutional right to health in Germany: A triumph of hope over evidence? *Health Economics, Policy and Law*.
Evans, David. 2003. Hierarchy of evidence: A framework for ranking evidence evaluating healthcare interventions. *Journal of Clinical Nursing* 12 (1): 77–84. https://doi.org/10.1046/j.1365-2702.2003.00662.x.
Fischer, Frank. 2003. *Reframing public policy*. Oxford: Oxford University Press.
Garrido, Marcial Velasco. 2008. *Health technology assessment and health policy-making in Europe: Current status, challenges and potential*. Copenhagen: WHO Regional Office Europe.
Gonzalez-Block, M.A. 2013. *Reflections on Health Policy and Systems Research embeddedness*. Presentation at Alliance for Health Policy and Systems Research at the Harvard School of Public Health, May 9.
Greenhalgh, Trisha, and Jill Russell. 2009. Evidence-based policymaking: A critique. *Perspectives in Biology and Medicine* 52 (2): 304–318.
Hammersley, Martyn. 2005. Is the evidence-based practice movement doing more good than harm? Reflections on Iain Chalmers' case for research-based policy making and practice. *Evidence & Policy: A Journal of Research, Debate and Practice* 1 (1): 85–100.

———. 2013. *The myth of research-based policy and practice*. London: Sage.
Hawkins, Benjamin, and Chris Holden. 2013. Framing the alcohol policy debate: Industry actors and the regulation of the UK beverage alcohol market. *Critical Policy Studies* 7 (1): 53–71.
Hawkins, Benjamin, and Justin Parkhurst. 2015. The 'good governance'of evidence in health policy. *Evidence & Policy: A Journal of Research, Debate and Practice* 12 (4): 575–592.
Howick, Jeremy. 2011. *The philosophy of evidence-based medicine*. Oxford: Wiley-Blackwell.
Immergut, Ellen M. 1992. *Health politics: Interests and institutions in Western Europe*. Cambridge: Cambridge University Press.
John, Peter. 1998. *Analysing public policy*. London: Continuum.
Koon, Adam D., Krishna D. Rao, Nhan T. Tran, and Abdul Ghaffar. 2013. Embedding health policy and systems research into decision-making processes in low-and middle-income countries. *BMC Health Research Policy and Systems* 11 (1): 30.
Lasswell, Harold Dwight. 1990 [1936]. *Politics; who gets what, when, how*. Gloucester: Peter Smith Publisher.
Lewis, Jenny M. 2003. Evidence-based policy: A technocratic wish in a political world. In *Evidence-based health policy: Problems & possibilities*, ed. Vivian Lin and Brendan Gibson, 250–259. Oxford: Oxford University Press.
Lin, Vivian, and Brendan Gibson. 2003. Introduction. In *Evidence-based health policy: Probelems and possibilities*, ed. Vivian Lin and Brendan Gibson, xvii–xxvi. Oxford: Oxford University Press.
Liverani, Marco, Benjamin Hawkins, and Justin O. Parkhurst. 2013. Political and institutional influences on the use of evidence in public health policy. A systematic review. *PloS One* 8 (10): e77404.
Lowndes, Vivien, and M. Roberts. 2013. *Why institutions matter*. Basingstoke: Palgrave.
Lukes, Stephen. 2005. *Power, a radical view*. 2nd ed. Houndsmills/Basingstoke: Palgrave Macmillan.
March, James G., and Johan P. Olsen. 1989. *Rediscovering institutions: The organisational basis of politics*. New York: The Free Press.
———. 2006. The logic of appropriateness. In *The Oxford handbook of public policy*, ed. Michael Moran, Martin Rein, and Robert E. Goodin, 689–708. Oxford: Oxford University Press.
Marmot, Michael G. 2004. Evidence based policy or policy based evidence? Willingness to take action influences the view of evidence – Look at alcohol. *British Medical Journal* 328: 906–907.
Nutley, Sandra, Isabel Walter, and Nick Bland. 2002. The institutional arrangements for connecting evidence and policy: The case of drug misuse. *Public Policy and Administration* 17 (3): 76–94.
Nutley, Sandra M., Isabel Walter, and Huw T.O. Davies. 2007. *Using evidence: How research can inform public services*. Bristol: The Policy Press.

Oliver, Kathryn, Simon Innvaer, Theo Lorenc, Jenny Woodman, and James Thomas. 2014a. A systematic review of barriers to and facilitators of the use of evidence by policymakers. *BMC Health Services Research* 14 (1): 2.

Oliver, Kathryn, Theo Lorenc, and Simon Innvaer. 2014b. New directions in evidence-based policy research: A critical analysis of the literature. *Health Research Policy and Systems* 12 (1): 34.

Parkhurst, Justin. 2016. Appeals to evidence for the resolution of wicked problems: The origins and mechanisms of evidentiary bias. *Policy Sciences* 49 (4): 373–393. https://doi.org/10.1007/s11077-016-9263-z.

———. 2017. *The politics of evidence: From evidence based policy to the good governance of evidence.* Abingdon: Routledge.

Peters, Guy. 2005. *Institutional theory in political science.* London: Continuum.

Peters, B. Guy. 2008. Institutional theory: Problems and prospects. In *Debating institutionalism*, ed. Jon Pierre, B. Guy Peters, and Gerry Stoker, 1–21. Manchester: University of Manchester Press.

Petrisor, B.A., and M. Bhandari. 2007. The hierarchy of evidence: Levels and grades of recommendation. *Indian Journal of Orthopaedics* 41 (1): 11.

Petticrew, Mark, and H. Roberts. 2003. Evidence, hierarchies, and typologies: Horses for courses. *Journal of Epidemiology and Community Health* 57 (7): 527–529.

Russell, Jill, Trisha Greenhalgh, Emma Byrne, and Janet McDonnell. 2008. Recognizing rhetoric in health care policy analysis. *Journal of Health Services Research & Policy* 13 (1): 40–46. https://doi.org/10.1258/jhsrp.2007.006029.

Sabatier, Paul A. 2007. *Theories of the policy process.* 2nd ed. Boulder: Westview Press.

Sackett, David L., William M.C. Rosenberg, J.A. Muir Gray, R. Brian Haynes, and W. Scott Richardson. 1996. Evidence based medicine: What it is and what it isn't. *British Medical Journal* 312: 71–72.

Sense About Science, and Academy of Royal Medical Colleges. 2013. *Evidence based medicine matters.* London: Sense About Science.

Smith, Katherine. 2013a. *Beyond evidence based policy in public health: The interplay of ideas.* Basingstoke: Palgrave Macmillan.

———. 2013b. Institutional filters: The translation and re-circulation of ideas about health inequalities within policy. *Policy & Politics* 41 (1): 81–100.

Starr, Mark, Iain Chalmers, Mike Clarke, and Andrew D. Oxman. 2009. The origins, evolution, and future of The Cochrane Database of Systematic Reviews. *International Journal of Technology Assessment in Health Care* 51 (Supplement 1): 182–195.

Stetler, C.B., J.A. Ritchie, J. Rycroft-Malone, A.A. Schultz, and M.P. Charns. 2009. Institutionalizing evidence-based practice: An organizational case study using a model of strategic change. *Implement Science* 4: 78. https://doi.org/10.1186/1748-5908-4-78.

Strassheim, Holger, and Pekka Kettunen. 2014. When does evidence-based policy turn into policy-based evidence? Configurations, contexts and mechanisms. *Evidence & Policy: A Journal of Research, Debate and Practice* 10 (2): 259–277. https://doi.org/10.1332/174426514X13990433991320.
Sutherland, Susan E. 2001. The evidence hierarchy. *Journal of the Canadian Dental Association* 67: 375–378.
Tuohy, Carolyn Hughes. 1999. *Accidental logics: The dynamics of change in the health care arena in the United States, Britain, and Canada*. Oxford: Oxford University Press.
Turchetti, Giuseppe, Enza Spadoni, and Eliezer Geisler. 2010. Health technology assessment. *IEEE Engineering in Medicine and Biology Magazine* 29 (3): 70–76.
Weiss, Carol H. 1979. The many meanings of research utilization. *Public Administration Review* 39 (5): 426–431.
———. 1991. Policy research: Data, ideas, or arguments. In *Social sciences and modern states: National experiences and theoretical crossroads*, ed. Peter Wagner, Carol Hirschon Weiss, Björn Wittrock, and Hellmut Wollmann, 307–332. Cambridge: Cambridge University Press.
Whitehead, Margaret. 1991. The concepts and principles of equity and health. *Health Promotion International* 6 (3): 217–228. https://doi.org/10.1093/heapro/6.3.217.
Wright, John S.F., Jayne Parry, and Jonathan Mathers. 2007. 'What to do about political context?' Evidence synthesis, the New Deal for Communities and the possibilities for evidence-based policy. *Evidence & Policy: A Journal of Research, Debate and Practice* 3 (2): 253–269.
Young, Iris Marion. 2000. *Inclusion and democracy*. Oxford: Oxford University Press.

Open Access This chapter is licensed under the terms of the Creative Commons Attribution 4.0 International License (http://creativecommons.org/licenses/by/4.0/), which permits use, sharing, adaptation, distribution and reproduction in any medium or format, as long as you give appropriate credit to the original author(s) and the source, provide a link to the Creative Commons license and indicate if changes were made.

The images or other third party material in this chapter are included in the chapter's Creative Commons license, unless indicated otherwise in a credit line to the material. If material is not included in the chapter's Creative Commons license and your intended use is not permitted by statutory regulation or exceeds the permitted use, you will need to obtain permission directly from the copyright holder.

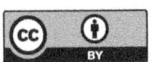

CHAPTER 2

The Many Meanings of Evidence: A Comparative Analysis of the Forms and Roles of Evidence Within Three Health Policy Processes in Cambodia

Helen Walls, Marco Liverani, Kannarath Chheng, and Justin Parkhurst

This chapter presents an edited version of a paper first published as:
Walls, H., M. Liverani, K. Chheng, and J. Parkhurst. 2017. The many meanings of evidence: A comparative analysis of the forms and roles of evidence within three health policy processes in Cambodia. *Health research policy and systems* 15 (1): 95.

H. Walls (✉) • M. Liverani
London School of Hygiene and Tropical Medicine, London, UK
e-mail: helen.walls@lshtm.ac.uk; marco.liverani@lshtm.ac.uk

K. Chheng
National Institute of Public Health, Cambodia, UK
e-mail: ckannarath@niph.org.kh

J. Parkhurst
London School of Economics and Political Science, London, UK
e-mail: j.parkhurst@lse.ac.uk

© The Author(s) 2018
J. Parkhurst et al. (eds.), *Evidence Use in Health Policy Making*,
International Series on Public Policy,
https://doi.org/10.1007/978-3-319-93467-9_2

Introduction

In this chapter, we investigate the evidence perceived to be relevant to policy decisions for three contrasting health policy examples in Cambodia – tobacco control, HIV/AIDS and performance-based salary incentives. These cases allow us to examine the ways that policy relevant evidence may differ given the framing of the issue and the broader institutional context in which evidence is considered.

It is widely agreed, including within the global health community, that data and evidence are essential to inform policy formulation and implementation (Lavis et al. 2004; Katikireddi et al. 2011; Macdonald and Atkinson 2011; Franklin and Budenholzer 2009). However the rhetoric of evidence-based policy – one based on the assumption that research is objective or unbiased, and its uptake is *a priori* positive, with particular emphasis given to pieces of evidence classified at the top of so-called 'hierarchies of evidence' – has long been critiqued by social science scholars (c.f. Oliver et al. 2014a, b; Cairney 2015; Cairney et al. 2016; Wesselink et al. 2014; Guyatt et al. 2008; Tunis et al. 2003; Liverani et al. 2013; Smith 2013a; Smith and Joyce 2012; Smith 2014; Hawkins and Parkhurst 2016). For example, Weiss (1990) has argued that research alone 'is almost never convincing or comprehensive enough to be the sole source of political advice', and 'there are always issues that research doesn't cover'. Increasingly policy-studies scholars have explored aspects of the political system that may shape when, how and the types of evidence used within policymaking (Cairney 2015). These can include both how political *institutions* (such as formal structures, and less formal rules and norms) (Lowndes and Roberts 2013) and how key *ideas* (including the way that issues are framed and understood) influence which types of evidence appear to be relevant for, and are used within, different policy processes (Smith 2013a; Shiffman and Smith 2007; Parkhurst 2012).

However, as described by Oliver et al. (2014a), little empirical analysis has been undertaken of the processes or impact of evidence use in policy and the way that research and policy processes interact. This paper seeks to help address this gap, through a comparative examination of the role that institutional and ideational factors play in shaping evidence use for three contrasting health policy decisions within a single country context. Specifically this paper presents findings from research conducted in Cambodia, where the Ministry of Health (MOH), like many government departments in countries elsewhere (Cabinet Office 1999; Government Office for Science 2012; DEFRA 2011), has explicitly embraced the overarching language of using 'evidence-based' approaches to health policymaking. One example of this endorsement is in the country's second Health Strategic Plan (2008–2015), which defines priorities and goals for the entire health sector, highlighting the need "to strengthen and invest in health information system and health research for evidence-based policymaking, planning, monitoring performance and evaluation" (Ministry of Health 2008). In this context, our study aimed to examine and compare the ways evidence was discussed or used in three contrasting health policy areas – tobacco control, HIV/AIDS and performance-based financing (PBF) – in particular for PBF we focus on a widely-praised government midwifery incentive scheme (GMIS) that was introduced to increase deliveries at public health facilities.

Tobacco control represents a policy decision for which there is a long history of acknowledged corporate and governmental financial interests that have often attempted to influence how health-related evidence is used in regulatory policy-making (Bero 2003, 2005; Ong and Glantz 2000; Tong and Glantz 2007). HIV/AIDS, on the other hand, is an issue with strong donor and global interest, and which has seen policy ideas particularly shaped by global civil society movements and consensus (Parkhurst 2012; Schneider 2002; Buse et al. 2008; Doyle and Patel 2008). Finally, PBF tends to have much less external contestation or debate, but is largely seen as a more technical matter related to health economics, health service provision or health systems functioning (Mills 2014; Meessen et al. 2011). As such, these three examples provide useful ways to reflect on how the different institutional settings in which policymaking takes place may influence evidence use, including how interests and ideas of key actors within the differing institutional arrangements play out in relation to evidence utilisation.

Methods

The paper draws on findings from in-depth semi-structured interviews conducted in Cambodia in 2015 and 2016 with stakeholders from key health sector organisations, as well as a related documentary analysis. The interviews were undertaken as part of a wider research project examining political aspects of evidence use for health policymaking in multiple countries. In case-study countries, key informants were first asked questions about the systems and processes through which evidence was used to inform health policy broadly, followed by asking for multiple examples of recent health policy decisions that could be illustrative of different aspects of evidence use. In all countries we subsequently investigated evidence use within tobacco control policy – given the importance of tobacco use for health in virtually every country context, as well as the existence of both a well-established evidence base and a global policy framework (i.e. the World Health Organization's global framework convention on tobacco control). After consultation with local stakeholders, we then selected additional country-specific health policy decisions of interest or importance to enable comparative analysis. As noted earlier, this approach led to the selection of three examples in Cambodia: tobacco control, HIV/AIDS and performance-based financing.

Key participants were identified though purposive and snowball sampling strategies. In line with our approach, we first approached high-level policy makers likely to be knowledgeable about major policy developments across the entire health sector, and thus could provide a general overview of systems and structures in place to use evidence and advice on the selection of case studies. Subsequently, a scoping review of relevant documents (i.e. published studies and grey literature in the public domain such as policy documents and reports) was conducted to collect background information on each policy issue. This was followed by identification of individuals who could comment further on the use of evidence to inform the selected policy decision. We endeavoured to conduct interviews with people who represented a diverse range of perspectives for the health decisions investigated. In total, 26 participants were interviewed, including both government representatives as well as individuals representing influential stakeholders in the policy process, particularly from aid providers, non-governmental organisations, multi-lateral organisations, and local research institutes.

Interview guidelines focused on the following broad topics, which were tailored to the different roles of informants and the specific expertise or insights they would bring: (1) perceptions about the policy process, including the role of different actors and contextual factors; (2) the nature and source of evidence that was used to inform the policy decision; (3) the way in which evidence was presented and evaluated; (4) general views on institutional structures and practices of evidence use within the Cambodian health sector. Interviews were conducted face-to-face by the authors, recorded (if permission was given), and subsequently transcribed and coded into themes in an iterative process (Bourque 2004). Citations from interviews and documents are included in the presentation of results to illustrate key points and emerging themes.

Consent was obtained at the initiation of each interview, with respondents given options on levels of anonymity desired. Ethical approval to undertake the study was provided by the London School of Hygiene and Tropical Medicine; and research permission obtained from the Cambodia National Ethical Committee for Health Research (n. 0120; 06/05/2014).

Policy Studies Perspectives

It is now reasonably well-established that national policy contexts can vary considerably with important implications for evidence use. Yet even within a single country, the characteristics of evidence use for different health issues may also vary considerably. Previous work has made it clear that the political nature of policymaking means that there can be multiple competing interests and concerns at stake for any given policy decision – even within the health sector (Parkhurst 2017; Russell et al. 2008; Cairney 2015). This indicates that multiple pieces of evidence may be relevant or considered in the policy process, depending on the differing concerns at stake, rather than any single piece or body of evidence. Thus an important step in moving beyond an over-simplistic treatment of evidence use is to understand the differing interests of stakeholders holding varying power and influence over a given policy decision. Indeed, Cairney notes that there can be such contestation at each step of the policy process – from defining the problem, to deciding which evidence to generate (or presumably which evidence to consider), to choosing solutions (Cairney 2015).

Scholars have thus begun to apply a range of theories and concepts from the policy sciences to help deepen our understanding of evidence use given these realities. Pearce (2014), for instance, describes a 'mistaken consensus' that local climate policy can be based on emissions data, instead drawing out how ideas and arguments are also used, and needed to construct local policy responses. This view is similar to that of Wellstead et al. (2017), who argue that climate change adaptation science advocates are too narrowly functionalist in assuming that policies will change in response to feedback about climate change. Instead they argue that understanding policy changes in this area requires looking not just at the specific problems climate science identifies, "but also at the political and institutional factors that transform situations into problems and attempt to address them (p. 13)".

This shift away from thinking about policy problems as fixed, but instead to consider how issues become 'problematised' directly draws on the field of interpretive (or critical) policy studies, which considers the roles of rhetoric or discursive framing in shaping policy outcomes (c.f. Fischer 2003; Bacchi 2009; Stone 2002). It is not just climate science, however, which has seen such developments in analysis. In looking at health policy, Smith (2013a), for example, argues that it is the roles and interplay of ideas (and ideas about evidence) that can be critical to understand evidence use within differing health-related concerns (Wesselink et al. 2014).

The policy sciences have thus been increasingly applied to questions of evidence use in health policymaking and beyond. These perspectives allow consideration of the multiple interests and multiple bodies of evidence that are important to a policy decision, while further recognising the ways that institutional and ideational factors can lead to differing constructions of what evidence is seen to be appropriate to address any given interest in the first place – with institutional forms and ideas closely linked to the relative influence of different stakeholders in policy processes.

In this paper, we embrace this approach, applying ideas from new institutionalism to explore the competing or contrasting constructions of evidence use for a set of three differing health policy concerns in the setting of Cambodia. On the one hand, new institutionalism highlights the not just the structures in place that shape decision making processes and outcomes, but also the importance of rules and norms within organisations that guide actor behaviours or decisions (Lowndes and Roberts 2013; Peters 2005). The approach also expands the focus of analysis beyond classic comparisons of state bureaucracies or legislative forms to consider the nature of institutionalised forces directing policy-relevant action across a much wider set of organisational forms, including non-state bodies, collections of stakeholders, or contrasting elements within a government system.

Applying such an approach to the question of evidence use for health thus allows us to focus on multiple issues. First we can consider the power or influence different stakeholders have over policy processes based on their structural positions for a given policy issue – reflecting on how different bodies of evidence may be more or less relevant to given stakeholders with influence. This approach also, however, allows exploration of the institutional logics which those stakeholders possess (c.f. March and Olsen 1989, 2006) that further shapes uses and understandings of policy-relevant evidence. In order to achieve these goals we first provide an overview of the three policy areas addressed, followed by a description of the types of evidence seen to be applied or important in each case. This is then followed by our analytical section that applies this institutional and ideational lens to explore such questions.

One Country, Three Health Policy Issues

Tobacco Control

Tobacco smoking became increasingly prevalent in Cambodia in the 1990s when the country was recovering from its civil war. At this time, there emerged the presence of many transnational tobacco companies in the country, the most prominent of which was British American Tobacco (BAT). The need for foreign investment and lack of regulation of advertising at this time, was explicitly recognised by British American Tobacco (BAT) who described Cambodia as "an attractive and strategically important target" (Mackenzie et al. 2004). A 1993 BAT industry plan, for example, acknowledged that awareness of the relationship between smoking and morbidity/mortality would increase in Cambodia through the activities of the World Health Organization (WHO), but estimated that "the significant revenues generated by tobacco advertising [for the government] will, in the short term, delay anti-smoking initiatives until alternative forms of revenue are guaranteed" (Mackenzie et al. 2004). BAT's preferred option was reportedly to become a majority shareholder in a joint venture alongside local interests. Such an arrangement would presumably allow industry control of the composition of company board of directors and significant influence over corporation activities, whilst also encouraging a local stake in the corporation's success. BAT achieved this in 1995 (Mackenzie et al. 2004).

According to Mackenzie et al. (2004) there was also at this time, owing to the lack of regulation, huge scope for tobacco-control advertising and promotional activities (Mackenzie et al. 2004). Indeed, a 1994 survey of twelve main streets in the country's capital Phnom Penh recorded 49% of the advertising signs (8495 in total) were advertising tobacco products (Smith 1996).

HIV/AIDS

HIV/AIDS in Cambodia has a very different history to tobacco smoking. In the mid-1990s, Cambodia had one of the fastest growing HIV prevalence rates in Southeast Asia, with injecting drug use and commercial sex driving HIV transmission (Weiss and de Cock 2001). Adult prevalence peaked at approximately 2.0% in 1998 (Pean et al. 2005). Since then, a number of prevention and treatment programmes have been introduced, however, and the country's prevalence has reduced, to an estimated 0.7% in 2013 (UNAIDS 2015; Vun et al. 2014).

The response has been divided into three phases: in phase I (1991–2000), a nationwide HIV prevention programme targeted brothel-based sex work, introduction of voluntary confidential counselling and testing and home-based care, and peer support groups of people living with HIV emerged; phase II (2001–2011) was characterized by expanding antiretroviral treatment (covering more than 80% of the population) and continuity of care, linking with other health services, accelerated prevention among key populations at higher risk (entertainment establishment-based sex workers, men who have sex with men (MSM), transgender persons, and people who inject drugs), engagement of health workers to deliver quality services, and strengthening health service delivery systems; and phase 3 (2012–2020) aims to attain zero new infections by 2020 through sharpening responses to high-risk population groups, maximizing access to community and facility-based testing and retention in prevention and care, and accelerating the transition from vertical approaches to linked/integrated approaches (Vun et al. 2014). In recognition of the country's success in halting and reversing the spread of HIV (relating to the United Nations Millennium Development Goal or MDG 6), Cambodia was in 2010 presented with an MDG Award (UNAIDS 2010).

Performance-Based Financing, and the Case of the Government Midwifery Incentive Scheme

The final health issue we explored in relation to the use of evidence was that of performance-based financing (PBF), with specific discussion in interviews about the role of evidence in supporting the government midwifery incentive scheme (GMIS). In many low and middle-income countries, PBF is increasingly being used to redress particular aspects of health system underperformance, particularly the productivity and quality of healthcare providers. It involves offering incentives intended to redress underperformance, particularly high worker absenteeism, which is frequently observed in poorly funded public health systems with poor accountability (van de Poel et al. 2016). Support for PBF has spread rapidly in many countries in recent years (van de Poel et al. 2016). But whilst there is considerable enthusiasm for PBF policies, according to a Cochrane Collaboration review (2012) of pay-for-performance to improve the delivery of health interventions in low- and middle-income countries, the current evidence base is too weak to draw any general conclusions regarding effectiveness, with more robust and comprehensive study needed (Witter et al. 2012; van de Poel et al. 2016).

According to van de Poel et al. (2016), Cambodia was the first documented case of a low-income country to experiment with PBF of public health care. Since 1999, a variety of health programme funding of districts and facilities in Cambodia have been contingent on performance targets or have directly linked revenues to services delivered. The main PBF programmes implemented have specified performance targets relating to child vaccination, antenatal care, delivery in a public facility, and birth-spacing use. These funding arrangements have been intended to increase aspects of healthcare provision, and there has been considerable variation in the strength and conditions of the incentives offered (van de Poel et al. 2016).

The interviewees specifically identified the GMIS as a notable PBF policy, and described how the policy contributed to reducing Cambodia's high maternal mortality ratio (MMR) over recent years. The GMIS became operational nationwide in late 2007, following a joint *prakas* (directive) from the MOH and MEF to allocate government budget to the incentive payments (Ir and Chheng 2012). The UNFPA was considered to be behind the policy change, for example through supporting a High-Level Midwifery Forum in late 2005 that bought together representatives from several government departments. However it was the prime minister who reportedly 'gave the green light' for the policy to go ahead. Other stakeholders were not thought to have had much direct influence over this decision, and the Cambodian Midwives Council, for example, was established after the implementation of the GMIS.

The GMIS aimed to boost facility deliveries by motivating skilled birth attendants (or trained health personnel) to promote deliveries in public health facilities. It did this by providing midwives (and other trained personnel) cash incentives based on the number of live births they attended in public health facilities – USD15 for a live birth in a health centre and USD10 for a live birth in a referral hospital. The reason for the higher payment in a health centre than a hospital was to provide a stronger incentive for deliveries at health centres – the recommended facility for normal deliveries to be managed (Ir et al. 2015). According to the MOH's guidance, besides midwives, physicians and other trained health personnel can also receive these incentives when attending deliveries in public health facilities. Up to 30% of the incentives will be shared with other health personnel in the facility and eventually with other people such as traditional birth attendants (TBAs) who refer women to the facility for delivery (Ir and Chheng 2012). The number of deliveries is reported monthly by health facilities through the routine health information system. Based on the number of reported deliveries, incentives are disbursed quarterly to the facilities through public financial disbursement channels (Ir and Chheng 2012).

THE NATURE OF EVIDENCE USED

In this section we begin to describe and examine the reported differences in evidence use between the three policy areas. The evidence relating to each issue can be categorised in various ways, including by evidence topic (e.g., health, economic) or type (e.g. epidemiological, pilot study), which relate to the issue framing by key stakeholders, and the sources relied upon (e.g. global literature, national statistics, government survey). What is clear, however, is that no single uniform construction of policy relevant evidence was seen across cases.

Tobacco Control

Global evidence on tobacco harms were at this time considered well established, but local data on smoking rates were fairly limited. In the late 1990s, Cambodia had some small regional surveys of smoking prevalence, but it wasn't until 2005 that accurate nationwide prevalence data on tobacco use were available (Singh et al. 2009). In spite of a lack of local data on smoking, in May 2004 Cambodia signed the Framework Convention on Tobacco Control (FCTC), a global policy agreement that calls for a number of restrictions on tobacco advertising and promotion – restrictions which many global health authors present as 'evidence based' (Myers 2013; Rosen et al. 2013; Glantz and Gonzalez 2012). Many stakeholders interviewed noted the importance of the FCTC locally, as it dictated that the government could not engage with industry on developing tobacco control policy. However implementation of the elements of the convention were described as only occurring slowly or in limited ways, which interviewees suggested was due to industry influence.

For example, one independent health sector consultant explained:

The tobacco industry and lobby is massively powerful here. (IDI[1]-01, June 2014)

[1] IDI, In-depth interview

Another respondent, a senior civil servant in the MOH, explained:

We don't know exactly why the law is very slow to be approved. Probably this is also due to lobbying of tobacco corporations, but we don't have evidence to prove it. (IDI-10, August 2014)

This individual also noted that tobacco control did not appear to be a priority in the national health sector strategic plan.

The context of a deeply entrenched and powerful tobacco interest was also manifested in how respondents conceptualised the evidence that was relevant for moving tobacco control policies forward. A number of civil servants interviewed, for example, stressed the need to counter other evidence the tobacco industry uses to frame tobacco control in a way that suits industry interests. For example:

They [tobacco corporations] always complain that if we increase taxes, farmers will lose their job. So, you have to explain to the government that, if you increase taxes, the margin will not affect the industry. Also, we have to explain that farmers do not rely on one crop only, so reduced tobacco production will not significantly affect them. (IDI-06, June 2014)

Tobacco industry is powerful and has money. Some people are lobbied by tobacco corporations. They [tobacco corporations] have a lot of experience. They can approach friends or members of the family and get confidential information about policy making. Then, people that are lobbied create opposition at the inter-ministerial meetings. They often say that tobacco control will impact on the economy and farmers. (IDI-08, August 2014)

Respondents also emphasised the importance of making different evidence-based arguments to different actors. In particular, it was noted that the Ministry of Economy and Finance (MEF) needed different evidence regarding tobacco control to the MOH to try to convince it to support policy action. As one civil servant explained:

You have to find a way to convince people... also because policy is multisectoral. It's not that one minister decides. If you want to increase tax, this is not an issue of the Ministry of Health. We don't have the power to do this. We can do a smoke-free policy, but tax is under the Ministry of Finance. So you have to work closely with the Ministry of Finance. In Cambodia, when you talk to the Ministry of Finance, first you have you prove to them they can make more money... The industry can say 'oh if you increase taxes, you will lose revenue'. And you have to present evidence that increasing taxes is not a loss of revenue. (IDI-06, June 2014)

We explain to the government that an increase in tax does not change the overall volume of cigarettes that are sold in the market. The case of Thailand shows this. Why? Because smoking prevalence decreases, but population increases. Cambodia is the same. Smoking prevalence has gone from 49.6% to 42.6%, however the absolute number of smoking is always 2 million because population increased... and you have to tell the government these facts. So you have to do a lot of work with the government to prove this. And of course, the tobacco industry makes a lot of money. We cannot stop them. (IDI-06, June 2014)

This civil servant also explained how evidence from neighbouring countries was considered influential, as was the normative element of the FCTC.

Usually in Cambodia we present evidence or examples from ASEAN[2] countries. How is Vietnam doing? Thailand? Indonesia? Then, we also do international. But ASEAN is very important, also because we are approaching the ASEAN [Economic] Community in 2015, and member countries do not want to be left behind. (IDI-06, June 2014)

Overall, whilst many of the respondents spoke of the slow progress of tobacco control policy in Cambodia, the government has made substantial progress in tobacco control by banning the advertisement of tobacco products in 2011 as well as smoking in workplaces and public spaces in 2016 using sub-decrees. However it wasn't until April 2015 that the Cambodian National Assembly passed the country's first-ever law on tobacco control, which was ratified later the same month. The new law tackles tobacco from a variety of angles, including through import and sales restrictions, and bans on sales to minors and pregnant women (FCTC Implementation Database 2014).

HIV/AIDS

HIV/AIDS policy-making illustrates a radically different political context in which the utilisation of health policy-relevant evidence can be explored. The United Nations AIDS programme (UNAIDS) has stated that Cambodia has "used high-quality strategic information to inform a [successful] evidence-based response" (UNAIDS 2012); and interviews stood in dramatic contrast to those with stakeholders advocating for greater

---

[2] Association of South East Asian Nations.

tobacco control who expressed the need to develop or discuss evidence of financial impact (e.g. on farmers or the treasury) to justify policy action. Instead, in discussions of HIV/AIDS, whilst a variety of evidence types were clearly brought to bear, NGO and donor-organisation respondents discussed how it has often been epidemiological modelling and cost-effectiveness analyses (IDI-21, 19, May 2016) – forms of evidence more typically advocated by public health actors for priority setting – that were seen as important evidence to guide policy. One of the respondents spoke about how this approach should be replicated in other areas of health policy-making:

I would say for HIV/AIDS it's that way [evidence use more technical than in other areas of policy] every time. I feel like that's brilliant and the model of HIV/AIDS [should] be replicated to other disease, for example we still have a very high number of death among pregnant women, the baby, the infant. So why don't they learn from the HIV/AIDS program. (IDI-21, May 2016)

When interviewees were asked about the use of evidence within particular policy developments, a range of evidence types were described, in addition to epidemiological modelling and cost-effectiveness studies mentioned above. Other relevant evidence was said to include pilot studies, used for example to inform the development of a community-based testing approach implemented in 2013, where the HIV testing is performed by lay counsellors – volunteers from population groups at higher risk of HIV infection. National prevalence estimates and international evidence were also evidence types that were frequently mentioned, particularly with international evidence from other Southeast Asian countries, and particularly Thailand. The importance of international evidence may also reflect the strong role of donors in HIV/AIDS policy-making in Cambodia.

Yes they [policymakers] welcome [overseas evidence] in the HIV area. I don't know about the other area. They welcome to learn the best practice from the region. This week one [NGO] staff member. He joined the field in Bangkok. (IDI-20, May 2016)

Epidemiological modelling of future prevalence scenarios has been considered key to informing policy as to the prioritization and targeting of interventions, preparation of operational plans, budgets and resource mobilization efforts (11) (12), and cost-effectiveness analyses such as modelling has highlighted areas where technical efficiency might be improved. The National Centre for HIV/AIDS, Dermatology and STI (NCHADS) within Cambodia's MOH, which is responsible for the health sector response to HIV and other sexually transmitted diseases, has led the analysis, in collaboration with relevant departments and centres of the MOH, the National AIDS Authority and other government institutions, as well as health service providers, non-governmental and other civil society organizations, and development partners.

When asked about the reasons why HIV/AIDS policymaking stood out in terms of the use of what is more typically considered policy-relevant health evidence, respondents particularly spoke of the strong donor interest and support for HIV policy-making in Cambodia. They felt that this was key to driving the type of evidence being used in policy-making, and also the relatively well-functioning institutional entry points for such evidence, including here the relevant technical working groups (TWGs) of the MOH. One NGO respondent explained:

> *Yes it's different [the policy-making process for HIV/AIDS compared to that for other health issues]. I think this is because donor support, and I think the other thing is because of resource, donor support and resource. Resource, I would say financial resource and human capacity resource, let's say for HIV/AIDS they have more educated [staff] and they adhere to plan, they adhere to target and they target evidence and I feel like the government take that approach very well, participatory approach, it's very well, because it's an emergency situation but it is also in the situation where funding is allowing so that's why we feel like they are open.* (IDI-21, May 2016)

However there were downsides to a donor-driven approach also described, including in relation to siloed, non-integrated evidence gathering. When asked what could be improved, one interviewee explained:

> *Well I think it's coordination. Because there's basically the different donor programme, donors put all the evidence together. It sits on programmes that are... like some donors who are actually doing their own evidence, but not systematically led by the national programme and disseminated in a timely manner.* (IDI-19, May 2016)

Interestingly, while HIV/AIDS policymaking has at times been seen as controversial or contested in some countries, related to the highly stigmatised nature of HIV transmission in some contexts (Rankin et al. 2005; Mahajan et al. 2008), we found little evidence of this in Cambodia. Whilst stigma and discrimination towards groups at higher risk of infection (sex workers, men who have sex with men (MSM), transgender persons and people who inject drugs) were noted, these were perceived to be relatively low compared to in many countries elsewhere. Instead, one of the NGO respondents explained that in Cambodia policy-makers are relatively open – and increasingly so – to discussing these groups and considering evidence relating to these groups.

> *The policy-makers they are more open now... for HIV the policy maker they are more open and learn from the [experience of high-risk groups].* (IDI-20, May 2016)

The respondents from a key NGO also spoke at length about the effort made by the NGO to engage high-risk population groups in the policy-making process, particularly in regard to supporting representatives to speak at community meetings and at the MOH TWG meetings.

> *[The NGO] work to promote that involvement in the policy-making as well, not only [the NGO] but also civil society. But we try to involve the key representatives from each key population to enrol in the policy-making process... we use the number, we use the finding, we use the civil society. But also bring the key population to talk during the meeting is more powerful... So this is like an MSM person or a sex worker, an entertainment worker could stand and speak about their challenges and the law enforcement people they listen to this. They're part of the meeting. Everyone is part of the meeting... They also listen and sometimes they [describe] their challenges and you can see some improvement.* (IDI-20, May 2016)

Performance-Based Financing, and the Case of the Government Midwifery Scheme

In contrast to the evidence types seen as relevant for tobacco control and HIV/AIDS policy-making, when asked about evidence for policy-making in regard to PBF schemes generally, these schemes were described as reliant almost solely on evidence from pilot studies. Interview respondents spoke of various pilot schemes of PBF that had been run over the years in different districts and by different groups, often by non-governmental organisations (NGOs), but also in workplaces of NCHADS. The perceived dominance of pilots as an evidence type is likely due to specific PBF policies being scaled up based on a pilot, but such schemes are likely also informed by evidence from health economics more broadly (and indeed, from basic microeconomics) that incentives can achieve outcomes (Mankiw and Taylor 2006). When pushed for further examples of evidence use in the PBF area, some respondents mentioned evidence from the Demographic and Health Survey, and also international evidence as informing the use of such schemes – but respondents didn't provide specific examples of such evidence. Some mentioned the low payment of midwives and the lack of incentives for women to deliver in health facilities as evidence for needed change.

> *I don't think anyone guided the government to design that policy. But it came clearly from many dialogues that the pay was not enough, that the arrangements did not encourage midwives to work in remote health centres, and did not encourage mothers to use health facilities.* (IDI-11, June 2014)

> *A few years ago there was a policy to put one midwife in each health centre and the midwifery incentive... Hun Sen acted on this, and the policy was implemented immediately and very effectively... the. trigger was the Demographic and Health Survey... it has quite a bit of impact, and there was a lot of pressure from the international community... it was a relatively 'easy fix', a simple solution.* (IDI-12, June 2014)

However, the dominance of pilots as an evidence type fits with observations from van de Poel et al. (2016) above, of Cambodia's pioneering role in experimenting with PBF of public health care, and also with one of our respondent's description of Cambodia as 'a country of pilots' (IDI-23, May 2016).

In contrast, however, there was also considerable discussion of that at times policy directives come from high levels of government – within the MOH, or as a decision made by the Prime Minister himself – and that in such situations evidence is perceived to be of limited importance. The GMIS was described as an example of this at times:

> *That [the GMIS] was an example of policy being changed by the government. It's the government's job, without any evidence.* (IDI-15, May 2016)

> *You know, in the United States the evidence has, as far as can tell, no effect on congress. But what happens is they pass laws and then health and human services when they're putting out the regulations or something, that's where the evidence comes in. Here it's more like everything at the congress level, even there is no, it doesn't get more rational as it comes down through the MOH... People have very set ideas about things and those aren't going to change no matter what evidence is put in front of them.* (IDI-22, May 2016)

You can present the evidence and present it passionately and you can present it unanimously when you are heard, but there's never really a proper policy dialogue. So saying well I could go and speak to the Ministry of Economy and Finance about that, we need extra money or we need to look at the budgets or perhaps we need to revise the [pre-service] training curriculum. You don't get that. (IDI-15, May 2016)

We don't even know who made it. There's a re-writing of history that claims the MOH thought about it but there was no evidence. I was here right after it started and know many people here when it started. At the time no-one was claiming the MOH invented it, so it came out of the MEF, the Ministry of Economy and Finance. It was actually hugely successful. (IDI-22, May 2016)

Another respondent from a donor agency was unable to name evidence in support of the policy, and instead described how he saw the policy process for the GMIS.

I think in Cambodia evidence [is not so important, rather] government want the community to deliver their baby at the health facility so the government just simply providing incentive to the health staff, community wide, so for delivery of one live birth delivery, they get $15.00 this is the decision by the government and government budget and then see if they implemented that. (IDI-17, May 2016)

This perception of success appears to come from data showing increasing facility utilisation for delivery and falling mortality rates nationally after implementation of the programme. Since then, the percentage of deliveries in public health facilities has increased substantially, from 29% in 2006 to 57% in 2011, and the MMR has declined substantially from 473 per 100,000 live births in 2005 to 206 in 2010 (Ir and Chheng 2012). Care, of course, is needed with interpretation of such evidence. A number of evaluations of PBF schemes such as the GMIS have been undertaken, and PBF policies have been credited with developments including increasing utilisation by the poor, decreasing total family per capita health expenditure and encouraging better management (Eldridge and Palmer 2009) – but drawing firm conclusions of causality can be problematic, particularly when such programmes have been implemented alongside other health sector reforms (Soeters and Griffiths 2003). One respondent further commented that the quality of evaluations undertaken is often poor.

INSTITUTIONAL FEATURES AND LOGICS OF EVIDENCE USE

The three policy areas presented show few similarities in how pieces of evidence were used in various aspects of policy making, despite all being discussed or undertaken within a single MOH, and within a broad policy environment in which 'evidence based policymaking' is rhetorically championed. In this section, however, we draw out some of the particular institutional and ideational features of the three health policy concerns that may help to explain these findings.

A starting point is to compare the institutionalised positions of influence of the key stakeholders in each case, to reflect on how the relevance of particular evidence types fit with the interests of such stakeholders. This can then be followed by considering any contrasting institutional logics that similarly might help explain differences in evidence utilisation. Such logics could either be direct thinking about which evidence is relevant and why (such as how public health actors explicitly embrace hierarchies of evidence at times), or they may be related to the overarching goals or expectations of the actors involved, which subsequently shapes their uses of evidence (such as when particular types of evidence more naturally align with or fit broader goals).

In the case of tobacco control, the historical influence of the tobacco industry appears particularly relevant, and the nature of contestation for this issue appeared to principally be framed in terms of financial implications of tobacco control. Our respondents described the financial importance of tobacco for the agricultural sector and the national economy as the paramount concerns for any policy change. Tobacco control were well aware of the need to present different evidence and frame the issue differently to address the concerns of the most influential stakeholders – with a particular distinction made between the health and economic evidence needed when speaking to policy-makers from the MOH and MEF, respectively. The need for taxation and other regulatory policy to be made outside the MoH illustrated how limited health-related evidence of tobacco harms could be in driving tobacco control policy forward on its own.

Evidence from neighbouring countries, and the FCTC, were said to be influential. But even so, and despite considerable progress, policy change in line with these was described as particularly slow, as too was the development of what were considered more appropriate forms of evidence to guide tobacco policy from a public health perspective, such as national smoking prevalence surveys. Despite global evidence on tobacco harms and increasing local data on smoking, it was the concerns regarding economic growth and the industry's entrenched interests and lobbying documented in our study and elsewhere (Mackenzie et al. 2004; Collin et al. 2004; Mackay 2004) that dominated the agenda. As such this significantly appeared to slow down the translation of the FCTC into local tobacco control policies; as well as the collection of, or action based on, forms of evidence typically seen as relevant to health promotion.

In contrast, the HIV/AIDS policy response in Cambodia developed in a rather different political context. With HIV/AIDS, there was no establishment of corporate interests, and little obvious financial interest at stake for any major stakeholders. Instead, the issue may have achieved a relatively high level of priority for policy action in Cambodia due to the attention and resources this issue has been accorded by donor agencies, and possibly related to this, the well-functioning TWGs of the MOH for HIV policy-making, as described by our respondents. The institutionalisation of donor influence is, in fact, reflected within the country's various strategic documents for guiding programme implementation – including the National Strategic Plan for HIV/AIDS, 2011–2015 (NSP III) and Cambodia 3.0, a strategy developed by the country's Ministry of Health to eliminate new HIV infections and congenital syphilis by 2020. Both are considered to be in line with the global targets and foci established by UNAIDS and the US PEPFAR programme (from which Cambodia is a recipient of funds) (PEPFAR 2015; UNAIDS 2015). These are highly technical global policy agencies, however, who routinely promote, or operate based around, particular forms of evidence types – embracing international discourses of evidence-based policy making. This may translate to the Cambodian context, particularly if there were no other strong interest groups to present alternative rhetoric or framing around the issue – and as such may have led to the use of evidence types in Cambodia more typically advocated by public health advocates in HIV/AIDS policy-making, and the observation of one NGO respondent that the National HIV/AIDS Centre is 'big on evidence' (IDI-25, May 2016).

Indeed, while in many countries the issue of HIV testing has been subject to debate or controversy – particularly around issues of disclosure or confidentiality of people living with HIV, and the challenges associated with addressing HIV in oft-stigmatised groups such as men who have sex with men, transgender people and sex workers – these concerns were considered by our respondents to have been relatively unimportant in Cambodia (even if admittedly seen as sensitive). That HIV/AIDS is an issue with social connotations in Cambodia perhaps explains the use of narrative evidence – stories of the lived experiences of marginalised groups – to influence policy-making. However, the relatively low level of moral contestation for this issue in Cambodia was noted – and used to explain the recent introduction of community-based rapid HIV testing (so-called 'finger-prick testing') by lay volunteer counsellors for high-risk population groups. Within this recent national policy, however, it was again evidence of effectiveness provided from a pilot study that could be seen to lead to policy change (KHANA 2014; Ministry of Health 2012).

The importance of pilots, however, was much more apparent, and described as the primary source of policy-relevant evidence for PBF. This was in contrast to tobacco policy appearing to require discussion of evidence of financial impact (linked to the influence of one set of interest groups), and HIV policy drawing particularly on epidemiological models and surveys (in line with norms and expectations of global health agencies). Again, however, we can look to the most influential stakeholders involved and their institutional logics to help explain the emphasis on pilots as a form of evidence in this case. Indeed, this helps to move away from the oft-criticised over-reliance on the idea that a single hierarchy of evidence can guide policy decisions, to instead consider the policy 'appropriateness' of particular forms of evidence (Parkhurst and Abeysinghe 2014; Dobrow et al. 2004; Young et al. 2002).

Unlike the previous cases, the GMIS policy appears to have had few stakeholders outside the government itself. It was reportedly made from the highest levels of the government, with some interviewees speculating that it was driven by the Prime Minister's office in particular in response to a feeling that some action must be taken to help achieve the maternal health millennium development goal by 2015. The power and influence in this case appeared to be particularly hierarchical, with decision making made through a planning and management orientation. Pilot studies, which examine feasibility of an intervention, are a first step in exploring novel interventions, novel applications of an intervention, or the feasibility of an intervention in a particular context when the effectiveness of that intervention may be context dependent (Leon et al. 2011). For this reason, they are often considered important evidence of effectiveness as well as feasibility within a particular context and for complex interventions, on the premise that cultural appropriateness of interventions is important and can shape outcomes (Bernal et al. 2009). As such, pilot studies have been described previously as particularly applicable in health services and health systems

Table 2.1 Characterisation of the institutional and ideational factors related to the health policy issue

Health policy area	Established dominant stakeholders	Institutional interests and logics	Nature of evidence used		
			Types	Topic	Source
Tobacco control	Industry, MEF	Financial importance of tobacco for agriculture sector and national economy	Regional surveys	Health	Local government,
			Epidemiological	Health	Global repositories
			Economic	Finance	Local sources
HIV/AIDS	International donors	Hierarchy of evaluation evidence; importance of achieving global targets	Epidemiological	Health	Global, local sources
			Economic	Finance	Local sources
			Pilot studies	Health	Local sources
			Narrative	Social	Citizens
PBF – GMIS	MoH, MEF, Prime Minister	Importance of achieving global targets; importance of achieving national implementation	Pilot studies	Health	Local (government, NGO)
			Epidemiological	Health	Local sources

research (Craig et al. 2013), but they also could be seen to be particularly relevant when a government has decided that wide-scale implementation of an intervention is a primarily objective at hand, such as achieving an MDG target through reducing the high maternal mortality rate.

In Table 2.1, we present a summary of these findings. In particular we highlight the stakeholders established to have dominant influence in each policy case, and their institutional interests and logics that help to explain the evidence said to be used by our interviewees.

Discussion

Despite a common use of the language of evidence-based policy making in the health sector, there are in fact many types of evidence which can speak to a variety of political concerns and mandates that play out in the policy process. Sometimes evidence use differs because the evidence needs differ to solve an agreed upon problem. At other times, there may not be any agreement on the nature of the problem, however, and as such it is features of power, interests, and framing that serve as important drivers shaping which evidence informs policy considerations. An institutionalist approach, however, can help to understand some of these dynamics. It can identify which stakeholders have established positions of power within differing health policy issues, linking their interests to the nature of evidence used. It can also reflect on the institutional logics of these stakeholders which further may influence when or how evidence is utilised.

For tobacco, large and expensive national prevalence surveys were considered necessary evidence for intervention, even given considerable evidence from smaller studies of a high prevalence of smoking in the country, and the irrefutable global evidence linking tobacco to numerous diseases and mortality. Such surveys, however, were needed because of a demand for evidence that could speak to the dominant concerns of financial impact and the logic that evidence was needed to illustrate economic impact, rather than any public health logic of evidence to show medical harm to the population. The importance of the ministry of finance is thus apparent in this case – illustrating both its dominant policy concern in terms of the economy, but also its logic of what forms of evidence are required to speak to that concern. Furthermore, it is of course critical to understand the historical influence and role of the tobacco industry in the country, which no doubt has played an important role in shifting the terms of tobacco policy to one of revenue.

In contrast, for the case of HIV/AIDS, the dominance of global donors in supporting this health issue, and the apparent limited contestation at a local level, appears to have led to the explicit embrace of epidemiological evidence that is widely held to be appropriate for HIV planning within the global health community. In the final case of PBF, however, it was the government that drove both the initiation and implementation of the policy response. This state-controlled process appeared to reflect a belief that national action must be taken to address an existing priority (in the form of a Millennium Development Goal). This in turn naturally led to a logic which saw relatively micro studies focussed on implementation to be the most policy-relevant. Although it is worth noting that in the case of the GMIS, some believed that evidence was not perceived as important at all, due to the policy being driven by higher level political authorities. Indeed, some stakeholders simply referred to the GMIS policy when asked for good example of the use of evidence because it was national action based around the 'evidence' that maternal mortality rates were too high – a much simpler logic of evidence informed policymaking whereby evidence of a problem is seen to justify widespread action, in contrast to more traditional health sector descriptions of evidence use being concerned with the effectiveness of interventions or possible alternative priorities or approaches.

Policy studies scholars would not be surprised, however, that powerful stakeholders (or 'vested interests') end up shaping the understanding of evidence, or which pieces of evidence are championed as relevant for policy making. This is perhaps most clearly illustrated in how evidence has been presented or selected by the tobacco industry in relation to policy-making debates (c.f. Smith 2013b; Ulucanlar et al. 2014; Tong and Glantz 2007; Bero 2005). For example, tobacco industry-funded studies have been shown to have misrepresented the association between second-hand smoke and CVD (Tong and Glantz 2007), or the evidence in support of standardised packaging of tobacco products (Ulucanlar et al. 2014). Tobacco interests have also emphasised evidence in support of the economic contributions of their product, whilst questioning the evidence suggesting that policy interventions are needed to protect health (Smith 2013b). HIV/AIDS, on the other hand, touches on issues of gender and sexuality, drug use and sex work, which often leads to it being seen as a highly morally-contested issue. However these did not appear particularly relevant in Cambodia, serving as a reminder that we cannot assume a health topic will necessarily exhibit the same political characteristics in different settings, even if such features are commonplace in other cases.

Conclusions

In the three contrasting case studies of evidence use in health policy-making examined in this study, evidence types – and their framing – were found to differ greatly, despite them taking place in the same country setting. The findings reiterate past authors' understandings that 'evidence' is not a uniform concept for which more is obviously better, or where a single model of 'evidence based policymaking' can prevail, but rather that different constructions and pieces of evidence become relevant given the politics involved in policy decisions, the nature of institutions involved, and the framing and conceptualisations of the issues themselves. Our comparative analysis helps to begin to trace out themes in linkages between the nature of contestation of health issues, the interests of established dominant stakeholders, and the logics by which those stakeholders operate – all of which work to shape which evidence is utilised or seen as policy relevant to inform health decisions. Whilst considerable further empirical research is needed in this area, this more nuanced understanding of evidence use may be of relevance to health policy-makers and others considering how to improve the role of evidence in health policy making.

Acknowledgements We are most grateful to the study participants for their contribution to the research.

REFERENCES

Bacchi, Carol Lee. 2009. *Analysing policy: What's the problem represented to be?* Frenchs Forest: Pearson Australia.

Bernal, Guillermo, María I. Jiménez-Chafey, and Melanie M. Domenech Rodríguez. 2009. Cultural adaptation of treatments: A resource for considering culture in evidence-based practice. *Professional Psychology: Research and Practice* 40 (4): 361–368.

Bero, L. 2003. Implications of the tobacco industry documents for public health and policy. *Annual Review of Public Health* 24: 267–288.

———. 2005. Tobacco industry manipulation of research. *Public Health* 120 (2): 200–208.

Bourque, L.M. 2004. Coding. In *The Sage encyclopedia of social science research methods*, ed. M.S. Lewis-Beck, A. Bryman, and T. Futing Liao. Thousand Oaks: Sage.

Buse, K., C. Dickinson, and M. Sidibe. 2008. HIV: Know your epidemic, act on its politics. *Journal of the Royal Society of Medicine* 101 (12): 572–573.

Cabinet Office. 1999. *Modernising government*. London: The Stationary Office.

Cairney, P. 2015. *The politics of evidence-based policymaking*. London: Palgrave Pivot.

Cairney, P., K. Oliver, and A. Wellstead. 2016. To bridge the divide between evidence and policy: Reduce the ambioguity as much as uncertainty. *Public Administration Review* 76 (3): 399–402.

Collin, J., E. LeGresley, R. Mackenzie, S. Lawrence, and K. Lee. 2004. Complicity in contraband: British American Tobacco and cigarette smuggling in Asia. *Tobacco Control* 13: ii104–ii111.

Craig, P., P. Dieppe, S. Macintyre, S. Michie, I. Nazareth, and M. Petticrew. 2013. Developing and evaluating complex interventions: The new Medical Research Council guidance. *International Journal of Nursing Studies* 50 (5): 587–592.

DEFRA. 2011. *Defra's evidence investment strategy: 2010–2013 and beyond*. London: DEFRA.

Dobrow, M.J., V. Goel, and R.E.G. Upshur. 2004. Evidence-based health policy: Context and utilisation. *Social Science & Medicine* 58 (1): 207–217.

Doyle, C., and P. Patel. 2008. Civil society organisations and global health initiatives: Problems of legitimacy. *Social Science & Medicine* 66 (9): 1928–1938.
Eldridge, C., and N. Palmer. 2009. Performance-based payment: Some reflections on the discourse, evidence and unanswered question. *Health Policy and Planning* 24: 160–166.
FCTC Implementation Database. 2014. Cambodia: New law on tobacco control passed. World Health Organization. http://apps.who.int/fctc/implementation/database/groups/cambodia-new-law-tobacco-control-passed
Fischer, F. 2003. *Reframing public policy*. Oxford: Oxford University Press.
Franklin, G.M., and B.R. Budenholzer. 2009. Implementing evidence-based health policy in Washington state. *The New England Journal of Medicine* 361: 1722–1172.
Glantz, S.A., and M. Gonzalez. 2012. Effective tobacco control a key to rapid progress in reduction of non-communicable diseases. *Lancet* 379 (9822): 1269–1271.
Government Office for Science. 2012. *Science and analysis assurance review of the Department for Work and Pensions*. London: Department for Business, Innovation and Skills.
Guyatt, G.H., A.D. Oxman, G.E. Vist, R. Kunz, Y. Falck-Ytter, P. Alonso-Coello, and H.J. Schünemann. 2008. GRADE: An emerging consensus on rating quality of evidence and strength of recommendations. *BMJ* 336: 924–926.
Hawkins, B., and J. Parkhurst. 2016. The 'good governance' of evidence in health policy. *Evidence & Policy* 12 (4): 575–592.
Ir, P., and K. Chheng. 2012. *Evaluation of Government Midwifery Incentive Scheme in Cambodia: An exploration of the scheme effects on institutional deliveries and health system*. Phnom Penh: Health System Development Support Unit, National Institute of Public Health.
Ir, P., C. Korchais, K. Chheng, D. Horemans, W. van Damme, and B. Meessen. 2015. Boosting facility deliveries with results-based financing: A mixed-methods evaluation of the government midwifery incentive scheme in Cambodia. *BMC Pregnancy and Childbirth* 15 (170): 170.
Katikireddi, S., M. Higgins, L. Bond, C. Bonell, and S. Macintyre. 2011. How evidence based is English public health policy? *BMJ* 343: d7310.
KHANA. 2014. *Peer-provided HIV testing and counselling for key populations in Cambodia: Lessons learned and ways forward*. Phnom Penh: KHANA.
Lavis, J.N., F.B. Posada, A. Haines, and E. Osei. 2004. Use of research to inform public policymaking. *Lancet* 364 (9445): 1615–1621.
Leon, A.C., L.L. Davis, and H.C. Kraemer. 2011. The role and interpretation of pilot studies in clinical research. *Journal of Psychiatric Research* 45 (5): 626–629.
Liverani, M., B. Hawkins, and J.O. Parkhurst. 2013. Political and institutional influences on the use of evidence in public health policy. A systematic review. *PLoS One* 8 (10): e77404.

Lowndes, V., and M. Roberts. 2013. *Why institutions matter: The new institutionalism in political science*. Basingstoke: Palgrave Macmillan.

Macdonald, I.A., and R. Atkinson. 2011. Public health initiatives in obesity prevention: The need for evidence-based policy. *International Journal of Obesity* 35: 463.

Mackay, J.M. 2004. The tobacco industry in Asia: Revelations in the corproate documents. *Tobacco Control* 13: ii1–ii3.

Mackenzie, R., J. Collin, C. Sopharo, and Y. Sopheap. 2004. "Almost a role model of what we would like to do everywhere": British American Tobacco in Cambodia. *Tobacco Control* 13: ii112–ii117.

Mahajan, A.P., J.N. Sayles, V.A. Patel, R.H. Remien, D. Ortiz, G. Szekeres, and T.J. Coates. 2008. Stigma in the HIV/AIDS epidemic: A review of the literature and recommendations for the way forward. *AIDS* 22: S67–S79.

Mankiw, N.G., and M.P. Taylor. 2006. *Microeconomics*. Thomson Learning.

March, J.G., and J.P. Olsen. 1989. *Rediscovering institutions: The organisational basis of politics*. New York: The Free Press.

———. 2006. The logic of appropriateness. In *The Oxford handbook of public policy*, ed. Michael Moran, Martin Rein, and Robert E. Goodin, 689–708. Oxford: Oxford University Press.

Meessen, B., A. Soucat, and C. Sekabaraga. 2011. Performance-based fnancing: Just a donor fad or a catalyse towards comprhensive health-care reform? *Bulletin of the World Health Organization* 89 (2): 153–156.

Mills, A. 2014. Health care systems in low- and middle-income countries. *New England Journal of Medicine* 370: 552–557.

Ministry of Health. 2008. Health Strategic Plan 2008–2015. Ministry of Health.

———. 2012. Standard operating procedures for HIV testing and counseling (HTC). Ministry of Health.

Myers, M.L. 2013. The FCTC's evidence-based policies remain a key to ending the tobacco epidemic. *Tobacco Control* 22: i45–i46.

Oliver, K., S. Innvar, T. Lorenc, J. Woodman, and J. Thomas. 2014a. A systematic review of barriers to and facilitators of the use of evidence by policymakers. *BMC Health Services Research* 14 (1): 2.

Oliver, K., T. Lorenc, and S. Innvaer. 2014b. New directions in evidence-based policy research: A critical analysis of the literature. *Health Research Policy and Systems* 12 (1): 34.

Ong, E.K., and S.A. Glantz. 2000. Tobacco industry efforts subverting Internatonal Agency for Research on Cancer's second-hand smoke study. *The Lancet* 355 (9211): 1253–1259.

Parkhurst, J.O. 2012. Framing, ideology and evidence: Uganda's HIV success and the development of PEPFAR's 'ABC' policy for HIV prevention. *Evidence & Policy* 8 (1): 17–36.

———. 2017. *The politics of evidence: from evidence based policy to the good governance of evidence*. Abingdon: Routledge.
Parkhurst, J.O., and S. Abeysinghe. 2014. What constitutes 'good' evidence for public health and social policy making? From hierarchies to appropriatness. *Social Epistemology Review and Reply Collective* 3 (10): 40–52.
Pean, P., S. Vong, M. Kato, V.S. Leng, and C.V. Mean. 2005. A new strategy for CD4 T-cell monitoring of HIV-positive patients at remote facilities in Cambodia [letter]. *AIDS* 19 (18): 2184–2185.
Pearce, Warren. 2014. Scientific data and its limits: Rethinking the use of evidence in local climate change policy. *Evidence & Policy: A Journal of Research Debate and Practice* 10 (2): 187–203.
PEPFAR. 2015. Cambodia country operational plan. www.pepfar.gov/countries/cop/240124.htm
Peters, Guy. 2005. *Institutional theory in political science*. London: Continuum.
Rankin, W.W., S. Brennan, E. Schell, J. Laviwa, and S.H. Rankin. 2005. The stigma of being HIV-positive in Africa. *PLoS Medicine* 2 (8): e247.
Rosen, L., E. Rosenberg, M. McKee, S. Gan-Noy, D. Levin, E. Mayshar, et al. 2013. A framework for developing an evidence-based, comprehensive tobacco control program. *Health Research Policy and Systems* 8: 17.
Russell, J., T. Greenhalgh, E. Byrne, and J. McDonnell. 2008. Recognising rhetoric in health care policy analysis. *Journal of Health Services Research and Policy* 13 (1): 40.
Schneider, H. 2002. On the fault-line: The politics of AIDS policy in contemporary South Africa. *African Studies* 61 (1): 145.
Shiffman, J., and S. Smith. 2007. Generation of political priority for global health initiatives: A framework and case study of maternal mortality. *The Lancet* 370 (13): 1370.
Singh, P.N., D. Yel, S. Sin, S. Khieng, J. Lopez, J. Job, L. Ferry, and S. Knutsen. 2009. Tobacco use among adults in Cambodia: Evidence for a tobacco epidemic among women. *Bulletin of the World Health Organization* 87: 905–912.
Smith, M. 1996. Advertising in Cambodia. *Tobacco Control* 5: 66–68.
Smith, K.E. 2013a. *Beyond evidence based policy in public health*. Basingstoke: Palgrave Macmillan.
———. 2013b. Understanding the influence of evidence in public health policy: What can we learn from the 'tobacco wars'? *Social Policy & Administration* 47 (4): 382–398.
———. 2014. The politics of ideas: The complex interplay of health inequalities research and policy. *Science and Public Policy* 41 (5): 561–574.
Smith, K., and K.E. Joyce. 2012. Capturing complex realities: Understanding efforts to achieve evidence-based policy and practice in public health. *Evidence and Policy* 8: 59–80.

Soeters, R., and F. Griffiths. 2003. Improving government health services through contract management: A case from Cambodia. *Health Policy and Planning* 18 (1): 74–83.

Stone, D. 2002. *Policy paradox: The art of political decision-making*. London: W.W. Norton & Company.

Tong, E.K., and S.A. Glantz. 2007. Tobacco industry efforts undermining evidence linking secondhand smoke with cardiovascular disease. *Circulation* 116: 1845–1854.

Tunis, S.R., D.B. Stryer, and C.M. Clancy. 2003. Practical clinical trials increasing the value of clinical research for decision making in clinical and health policy. *JAMA* 290 (12): 1624–1632.

Ulucanlar, S., G.J. Fooks, J.L. Hatchard, and A.B. Gilmore. 2014. Representation and misrepresentation of scientific evidence in contemporary tobacco regulation: A review of tobacco industry submissions to the UK government consultation on standardised packaging. *PLoS Medicine* 11 (3): e1001629.

UNAIDS. 2010. Cambodia takes MDG prize for excellence in its AIDS response. http://www.unaids.org/en/resources/presscentre/featurestories/2010/september/20100920fsmdgcamboda-award/

———. 2012. Case study: The Royal Government of Cambodia at the forefront in applying new investment approach. In *Thirty-first meeting*. Geneva: UNAIDS.

———. 2015. Cambodia country progress report: Monitoring progress towards the 2011 UN political declaration on HIV and AIDS.

van de Poel, E., G. Flores, P. Ir, and O. O'Donnell. 2016. Impact of performance-based financing in a low-resource setting: A decade of experience in Cambodia. *Health Economics* 25: 688–705.

Vun, M.C., M. Fujita, T. Rathavy, M.T. Eang, S. Sopheap, S. Sovannarith, C. Chhorvann, L. Vanthy, O. Sopheap, E. Welle, L. Ferradini, C. Sedtha, S. Bunna, and R. Verbruggen. 2014. Achieving universal access and moving towards elimination of new HIV infections in Cambodia. *Journal of the International AIDS Society* 17 (1): 18905.

Weiss, C. 1990. Policy research: Data, ideas or arguments? In *Social science and modern states*, ed. P. Wagner et al. Cambridge: Cambrdge University Press.

Weiss, H.A., and K.M. de Cock. 2001. The global epidemiology of HIV/AIDS. *Tropical Medicine & International Health* 5 (7): A3–A9.

Wellstead, A., and M. Howlett. 2017. Structural-functionalism redux: Adaptation to climate change and the challenge of a science-driven policy agenda. *Critical Policy Studies* 11 (4): 391–410.

Wesselink, A., C. Colebatch, and W. Pearce. 2014. Evidence and policy: Discourses, meanings and practices. *Policy Sciences* 47 (4): 339–344.

Witter, S., A. Fretheim, F. Kessy, and A. Lindahl. 2012. Paying for performance to improve the delivery of health interventions in low- and middle-income countries. *Cochrane Database of Systematic Reviews* 2: CD007899.

Young, K., D. Ashby, A. Boaz, and L. Grayson. 2002. Social science and the evidence-based policy movement. *Social Policy & Society* 1 (3): 215–224.

Open Access This chapter is licensed under the terms of the Creative Commons Attribution 4.0 International License (http://creativecommons.org/licenses/by/4.0/), which permits use, sharing, adaptation, distribution and reproduction in any medium or format, as long as you give appropriate credit to the original author(s) and the source, provide a link to the Creative Commons license and indicate if changes were made.

The images or other third party material in this chapter are included in the chapter's Creative Commons license, unless indicated otherwise in a credit line to the material. If material is not included in the chapter's Creative Commons license and your intended use is not permitted by statutory regulation or exceeds the permitted use, you will need to obtain permission directly from the copyright holder.

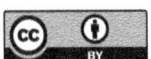

CHAPTER 3

The Role of Evidence in Nutrition Policymaking in Ethiopia: Institutional Structures and Issue Framing

Helen Walls, Deborah Johnston, Elisa Vecchione, Abdulfatah Adam, and Justin Parkhurst

---

This chapter presents a version of a paper subsequently published as:
Walls, Helen, Deborah Johnston, Elisa Vecchione, Abdulfatah Adam, and Justin Parkhurst. 2018. "The Role of evidence in nutrition policymaking in Ethiopia: institutional structures and issue framing." *Development Policy Review.* https://doi.org/10.1111/dpr.12385.

H. Walls (✉) • E. Vecchione
London School of Hygiene and Tropical Medicine, London, UK
e-mail: Helen.walls@lshtm.ac.uk; e.vecchione@ucl.ac.uk

D. Johnston
SOAS University of London, London, UK
e-mail: dj3@soas.ac.uk

A. Adam
University of Copenhagen, Copenhagen, Denmark
e-mail: abad@sund.ku.dk

J. Parkhurst
London School of Economics and Political Science, London, UK
e-mail: j.parkhurst@lse.ac.uk

© The Author(s) 2018
J. Parkhurst et al. (Eds.), *Evidence Use in Health Policy Making*, International Series on Public Policy, https://doi.org/10.1007/978-3-319-93467-9_3

INTRODUCTION

Malnutrition is the single greatest contributor to the global burden of morbidity and mortality, affecting one in three people worldwide, with the majority of cases arising in low- and middle-income countries (LMICs) (Kassebaum 2014; Bhutta and Salam 2012). Initiatives to address this include including the 2025 World Health Assembly nutrition targets, the Sustainable Development Goal target of ending all forms of malnutrition by 2030, and global initiatives such as the Scaling Up Nutrition movement (Gillespie et al. 2013; International Food Policy Research Institute 2015).

Nutrition policy involves collaboration between the agriculture, health and environment sectors (c.f. Gillespie et al. 2013; Mendis 2010; Bonita et al. 2013; Reinhardt and Fanzo 2014). However, this adds considerable complexity to the implementation of effective programmes (Balarajan and Reich 2016), with need for better understanding of the linkages between sectors to improve nutritional outcomes. Several countries have achieved considerable success with addressing malnutrition in recent years (WHO 2013). However, global progress has generally been slow, with many countries failing to achieve nutrition targets (International Food Policy Research Institute 2015; Roberto et al. 2015; Heaver 2005; Lachat et al. 2013).

Achieving nutrition goals requires policy action at the national level. This raises questions about why or how relevant policy change may come about within different country settings. As Chap. 1 in this volume discusses, the global health community has increasingly embraced the language of 'evidence-based policy' (or 'evidence-informed policy') to describe the ways in which research evidence provides clear policy solutions to health policy concerns. However, several case studies, including from LMICs, have illustrated the difficulties in applying these ideas in practice. Nabyonga-Orem and Mijumbi (Nabyonga-Orem and Mijumbi 2015), for instance, reflected on the Ugandan experience of evidence utilisation, stating:

> although there is a general agreement on the benefits of evidence informed health policy development given resource constraints especially in low-income countries, the definition of what evidence is, and what evidence is suitable to guide decision-making is still unclear. (p. 285)

Similarly, Shiffman (2006) found that, in aid-recipient countries, donor funding for communicable diseases did not reflect the evidence base on disease burden, which offer a rationale for prioritising policy action. Rather than there being any single process by which evidence is applied in policy development, complex political dynamics and normative ideas shape processes of evidence use (c.f. Nutley et al. 2007). The political nature of decision-making involves multiple contested interests, making it difficult to achieve agreement on which policy problems and policy outcomes should be prioritised (Parkhurst 2017). This has led Smith (2013) to argue that it more important to analyse ideas (about evidence) and how they shape policy rather than assuming evidence itself will have any consistent influence.

Ideas about evidence use exist collectively and are embedded within particular institutional norms and practices. Policy decision-making behaviours within institutions can thus be shaped and constrained by so-called 'logics of appropriateness' that serve to direct ways of working or thinking for individuals within particular institutional arrangements (Lowndes and Roberts 2013; March and Olsen 1984; Peters 2008). While the dominant way of thinking about evidence use to inform decisions in the global health community can therefore be conceptualised as one particular institutional logic, the multi-sectoral nature of nutrition policymaking raises questions about how health sector actors can engage with stakeholders that have differing priorities, and potentially different logics of evidence use.

Studying the process of nutrition policy formation can thus provide a useful lens to explore these issues of the roles and use of evidence in the context of multi-sectoral nutrition policy planning. Our perspective focusses primarily on the health sector yet our findings highlight different sectorial perspectives and logics in regard to a particular policy formulation. This chapter focuses on a case study of Ethiopia, which provides a unique example of the challenging nature of multi-sectoral nutrition policy-making, even with strong coordinating infrastructure. Although the government of Ethiopia implemented a National Nutrition Programme (NNP) in 2008 and integrated it with the overarching national strategic framework, the Growth and Transformation Plan 2010/11–2014/15 (GTP I) (Federal Democratic Republic of Ethiopia 2011), problems with multi-sectoral working have been acknowledged (Government of Federal Democratic Republic of Ethiopia 2016, pp. 20–21). Consequently, the structure for multi-sectoral working was strengthened in the third NNP, NNP-II (2016–2020) (Government of the Federal Democratic Republic of Ethiopia 2016) and in the GTP- II, 2015/16–2019/20 (Ethiopia 2016).

This chapter illustrates the challenges with nutrition policymaking expressed by health sector stakeholders in interviews undertaken in December 2014. It examines the problems observed in multi-sectoral working from the health sector perspective. Furthermore, it uses these – reflections on the likely success of NNP-II. It suggests that although Ethiopia has made progress with the coherence of its strategic planning, tensions remain with inter-sectoral alignment of nutrition concerns. The paper highlights three issues which we argue remain unresolved: the framing of nutrition in Ethiopia; the development of internal nutrition logics in complementary sectors; and the remaining gaps in the evidence base.

The Case of Ethiopia

Ethiopia has historically faced nutrition challenges in regard to drought and famine, and undernutrition remains a significant challenge in the country today (Hazards and Vulnerability Research Institute 2014). Nearly 8 million people in Ethiopia are considered to be chronically food insecure and thus supported through a national social protection programme, the 'Productive Safety Net Programmes' (aiming to "enable the rural poor facing chronic food insecurity to resist shocks, create assets and become food self-sufficient"), through multi-annual transfers of food and cash (World Food Programme 2017). Recent (2016) USAID figures indicate that 10 million more people are in need of emergency food assistance (USAID 2016).

Increasingly, however, Ethiopia is also facing problems of overweight, obesity and related non-communicable diseases (NCDs) (Zello 2015; Tebekaw et al. 2014), although this is mainly confined to urban settings. The 2011 Demographic and Health Survey estimated 6% of women (aged 15–49 years) to be overweight or obese (Ethiopia Central Statistical Agency and ICF International 2012); a low prevalence by global standards (Malik et al. 2013). Yet, the 'double burden' of co-existing issues of underweight and overweight presents a new and significant challenge for Ethiopian nutrition policy (Walls et al. 2016b).

Ethiopia's political-administrative structures for nutrition policy have been shaped by its history of cyclical drought and famines, civil conflict and insurgency (Keller 1992; Webb and von Braun 1994) and, more recently food insecurity resulting from increasing climate variability (Kassie et al. 2013, 2014). Today, the Ethiopian Public Health Institute (EPHI) is the advisory body mandated to provide research and evidence to inform nutrition policy in the country.

Historically, nutrition policy in Ethiopia was focused on acute or emergency food shortages (Embassy of the Federal Democratic Republic of Ethiopia 2016; Federal Democratic Republic of Ethiopia 1996). However, in recent years there have been efforts to establish broader and more systematic policy responses to nutrition driven by the need to address the Millennium Development Goals (MDGs) (Benson 2005; Ethiopian Academy of Science 2013), and provided the basis for the 2008 National Nutrition Strategy (NNS) (Federal Ministry of Health 2008).

A more comprehensive nutrition policy has been prioritised by the central government in Ethiopia in recent years. Ethiopia's first National Nutrition Programme (NNP) 2008–2013 acknowledged the role of multiple sectors including health, agriculture, education, and social affairs in addressing population nutrition, creating the National Nutrition Coordination Body (2008) and the National Nutrition Technical Committee (2009) and chaired and co-chaired by the State Minister of Health and State Minister of Agriculture and Natural Resources respectively (Ministry of Health 2015). The revision of NNP (resulting in NNP-I (2013–2015)) endeavoured to address problems arising from this multi-sectoral approach (Government of the Federal Democratic Republic of Ethiopia 2013). To supplement multi-sectoral working, the government established the National Nutrition Coordination Body (NNCB) and the National Nutrition Technical Committee (NNTC), with the intention of coordinating and mainstreaming nutrition into various sectors.

In terms of nutrition-related outcomes, official documents point to substantial declines between 2000 and 2015 in the prevalence of maternal anaemia, stunting, underweight children, and in anaemia among children under-five (Government of the Federal Democratic Republic of Ethiopia 2016). However, the prevalence of wasting remained fairly static (p. 13) (Government of the Federal Democratic Republic of Ethiopia 2016).

Overall, however, high levels of malnutrition remain. Related to this, NNP-II found that most ministries "have lagged in mainstreaming nutrition into their sectoral strategic plans. (Government of the Federal Democratic Republic of Ethiopia 2016, p. 21)." Sectoral departments lacked an effective organisational structure to mainstream nutrition; sectoral plans were not always reshaped to include nutrition goals; sectoral nutrition plans were not allocated a budget; responsibilities and accountabilities were not clearly defined around shared goals; and finally, the mechanisms to capture nutrition-relevant data from all sectors were not developed (Government of the Federal Democratic Republic of Ethiopia 2016). The NNP-II aimed to improve this situation by three broad sets of actions: strengthening the NNCB and local coordination bodies; requiring ministries to establish new nutrition capacity; and establishing both new evidence and new evidence-based decision-making systems (Government of the Federal Democratic Republic of Ethiopia 2016).

To date, there has been only limited research conducted on Ethiopian nutrition policymaking; with little explicit consideration of the role of evidence. Nisbett et al. (2015) explored leadership in tackling child undernutrition in Ethiopia and identified external challenges influencing individual leadership in nutrition policy, including a lack of local-level knowledge, evidence and data to inform policy. In particular, the authors highlighted the 'siloed' nature of local knowledge and data collection and advocated for a need to "look at the bigger picture and answer the big research questions" (Nisbett et al. 2015, p. 41). Kennedy et al. (2015), on the other hand, examined the governance of nutrition policy, finding general agreement at multiple levels on the nature of the problem, but various challenges such as limited leadership, funding, coordination, and incentives for inter-sectoral collaboration (Kennedy et al. 2015).

This study extends earlier research and provides more evidence of some of the challenges documented above. By engaging with the specific theme of evidence use to inform policy decision-making for nutrition in a context of multi-sectoral planning, it focuses on a key issue that has been identified as constraining multi-sectoral coordination.

METHODS

The article draws on findings from 23 in-depth semi-structured interviews with stakeholders from key health sector organisations. The interviews were undertaken as part of a wider research project on the political aspects of evidence use for health policymaking in multiple countries Interviews focussed on key themes including: the structures and functions of evidence use within the Ethiopian health sector; the institutional mechanisms for evidence uptake; and investigation of the roles of evidence in influencing recent or important health policy decisions in the country; with a subset of five interviews also specifically exploring the theme of evidence use for nutrition policy. Interview data were combined with a documentary analysis of federal and relevant international strategies, plans and reports.

Key participants were identified though purposive and snowball sampling strategies. We endeavoured to conduct interviews with policy actors representing a diverse range of perspectives for the health decisions investigated. Participants involved senior and mid-level stakeholder representatives from a range of institutional types, including government (including from the Ministry of Health and Ethiopian Public Health Association), international donor agencies (including from UNICEF, Save the Children, the US Centers for Disease Control, and European Union), academic researchers and other independent non-for-profit groups (including from Addis Ababa University, the Ethipioan Academy of Sciences, and the Addis Continental Institute of Public Health), and corporate interests (including from the National Tobacco Enterprise).

Consent was obtained at the initiation of each interview, with respondents given options on levels of anonymity desired. Ethical approval was provided by the London School of Hygiene and Tropical Medicine; and research permission was obtained from the Ethiopian Public Health Institute. As part of the questioning about evidence use for health policymaking in Ethiopia more generally, respondents were asked for examples of particular health issues that could illustrate the application of the broader ideas and structures shaping evidence use. The respondents spoke about a range of issues, and nutrition was an important issue discussed by a number (5) of the respondents from a broad range of institutional types (government, academia and international donor agency), leading to further investigation into this issue and the analysis undertaken in this paper.

Analysis of interviews involved manual coding of key themes emerging from the interviews. This included reading the interview transcripts and recording key themes, and then cross-checking these themes through searches of key terms of emerging interest. To refine our understanding of the information from interviews, this information was then compared with and supplemented by that obtained from the documentary review.

In addition to the published academic sources cited throughout this paper, the documentary review included a set of unpublished sources related specifically to Ethiopia.

FRAMING OF NUTRITION

Despite wide embrace of the idea that evidence should inform policymaking, it has long been recognised that *policy-relevant* evidence is understood differently by different policy communities (c.f. Nutley et al. 2007; Parkhurst 2017; Weiss 1979). As such, it is important to consider how policy issues are framed and how this shapes which pieces of evidence, or what forms of evidence, are considered relevant. Unsurprising given its past famines, nutrition has historically been framed in Ethiopia as an acute or emergency issue. According to one interviewee, this focus could also be seen to affect the research agenda on nutrition in the country:

> *My impression is there is a lot of research especially on emergency nutrition... food shortage and acute malnutrition and that seems to affect a significant part of the population and it has been a constant focus for many NGOs and the government. So much of the research that I have seen is usually around this.* (IDI[1]-17)

As described above, many recent policy documents further illustrate the Government of Ethiopia's focus on undernutrition, with an emphasis on key population groups such as children and mothers. These policy documents have considerably less focus on nutrition problems linked to overweight. In the NNP-I (2013–2015), for instance, the word 'obesity' is mentioned once, in regard to its increasing prevalence in urban areas, while 'overweight' is not mentioned at all (Government of the Federal Democratic Republic of Ethiopia 2013). Yet our health sector respondents spoke frequently about a shifting conceptualisation in which nutrition as a chronic issue – particularly in regard to overweight/obesity – was of increasing importance in policy considerations:

> *We have a high prevalence who are underweight, but we also have overweight, which is coming... The MOH has already prioritised both under and over nutrition because you will be surprised, you know in Addis and in the other city, in Dire Dawa, you see overweight is also a problem.* (IDI-17)

Government policy documents such as the HSTP describe how risk factors for overweight, obesity and NCD, including physical inactivity and unhealthy diets, are widely prevalent in Ethiopia; and particularly in urban areas (Ministry of Health 2015). The NNP-II (2016–2020) (Government of the Federal Democratic Republic of Ethiopia 2016) has more information relating to overweight and obesity, and also includes an indicator on overweight women. However, no indicators relate to overweight children, and core goals and objectives remain focused on undernutrition. The perception of respondents was thus that any recent shift in research and evidence generation to focus on overweight/obesity and associated NCDs as

---

[1] IDI refers to in-depth interview, with anonymous numbers assigned.

described during fieldwork 2014, largely remained at odds with the national policy response; which was felt to only minimally address overweight and obesity in national strategies.

One potential explanation for this could be that global framings or conceptualisations regarding nutrition were being picked up in local discourses – even if it appears to a much lesser extent in existing policy. The international literature has increasingly in recent years linked undernutrition with overweight and obesity-related health issues, and there has also been a dominant discourse in the global health community on the need for more multi-sectorial and structural policy responses to addressing nutrition (Kanter et al. 2015; Ruel et al. 2013; Dangour et al. 2013; Garrett and Natalicchio 2011; World Bank 2013). Such a push would address the underlying causes of malnutrition. This framing was also identified in local interviews, with individuals in four separate interviews raising the issue.

> *It's now established, there are many studies which have proved this, people who have been affected by under nutrition during childhood in the first years of life, these are critical years, and … they will have a much higher risk of hypertension, overweight, obesity.* (IDI-17)

> *The MoH [is the main actor in recent nutrition policy] and the second we can consider the other actors for example other sector, actually the nutrition issue is not only for the health issue it is the concern of other sectors like agriculture, education, water, actually nine sectors are involved [in revising the NNP]… Nutrition is a multsectoral and multidimensional issue.* (IDI-23)

This thinking, however, was reflected in national documents as well. The HSTP, for instance, describes nutrition as a 'cross-cutting' issue (Ministry of Health 2015), and two of the five objectives of NNP-I and NNP-II relate to this emphasis on multi-sectoral action (Government of the Federal Democratic Republic of Ethiopia 2013). The *Situation Analysis of the Nutrition Sector in Ethiopia* also reflects this focus, with suggestions for greater multisectoral efforts, including a policy recommendation to 'revisit existing agricultural politics to make them nutrition sensitive with a clear result framework' (p. 85) (FMoH/UNICEF/EU Situation Analysis of the Nutrition Sector in Ethiopia: 2000–2015 2016).

There was a suggestion from interviewees that this view in Ethiopia of nutrition as a multi-sectoral issue may particularly have been influenced by the 2008 *Lancet* nutrition series, which happened to be launched in Addis Ababa. As respondents explained:

> *Nutrition is not only public health, it's many other aspects. Like even globally even if you look at [it] from the Lancet for example the cause of stunting only 20% is nutrition-specific the other is nutrition-sensitive which is not related health. So we are saying that nutrition is beyond the health.* (IDI-13)
>
> *So one of the issues is actually the fact it needs really multi-sectoral action, and that is a big challenge and I was there following the launch of that [Lancet] strategy....* (IDI-17)

CHALLENGES TO AN 'UPSTREAM' AND MULTISECTORAL APPROACH

The 'upstream/downstream' metaphor commonly used in public health captures concerns between paying attention to prevention versus treatment of health issues; with prevention about consideration of the causes of health problems (Dorfman and Wallack 2007). An upstream focus would address the more distal causes of the problem, sometimes described as the 'causes of the causes' (Marmot 2005), and with nutrition might be addressed through leveraging agricultural policy or larger political-economy drivers (Balarajan and Reich 2016). A downstream focus would be more proximal to the individual, focused perhaps on education and information, or provision of micronutrient supplements.

Whilst there may be a growing recognition and desire to respond to nutrition in an upstream or structural manner, policy interventions for nutrition globally have been described as traditionally focussing downstream – on potentially less effective, or less sustainable interventions (Walls et al. 2016a, b). Such interventions can more easily lend themselves to measurable (though not necessarily greatest) policy impact, and clearer evidence generation.

Our interviews identified criticisms of downstream approaches to addressing nutrition in Ethiopia, with one interviewee criticising the government for supporting a micronutrients approach, instead of 'an integrated dietary approach' which the respondent believed should start with food diversification and only rely on supplementation as a last resort (IDI-17). The first version of the NNP (2008–2013), launched prior to this report, gave little emphasis to the micronutrients approach. In fact, the National Food Fortification Programme was among the chief reasons for revising the original NNP (Government of the Federal Democratic Republic of Ethiopia 2013). Since then, food supplementation in the form of vitamin A for children under 5 and zinc supplementation for diarrhoea treatment had been implemented. In addition, legislation requiring salt iodization has been put in place (Government of the Federal Democratic Republic of Ethiopia 2013).

Food fortification is considered a means to rapidly address nutrition challenges. Some health actors expressed the view that the reasons driving policy action in agriculture differ to those in health, and this reflected a more general challenge of enacting structural policy changes when doing so requires engagement from other sectors, especially the agriculture sector – seen to be key to a multi-sectoral nutrition response.

If you look at the causes of under nutrition it easily goes outside the health system. So one is for example food security, food security is a question of having sufficient land productive...the main target for the MOH is to decrease mortality and you can't do that without addressing undernutrition. So I think it makes sense to give this assignment to the MoH but there should be also a way to give it more power so that's the whole idea... The only thing is the MoH should have more strong department and representatives from all ministries. (IDI-17)

One respondent, for instance, explained that the MoA mandate is to increase productivity, and that it is evaluated by this target rather than on the nutritional outcomes of its policies per se. (IDI 13). This reflects the focus of the first GTP, as previously described (Federal Democratic Republic of Ethiopia 2011).

The advice to the public from the agricultural sector – advice regarding promotion of economic aspects of agricultural production and not its potential to improve nutrition – was considered by respondents to be unhelpful from a nutrition perspective, and even in contradiction to advice from the MoH. Additionally, agricultural policy was considered not to be 'nutrition sensitive'.

[Much agricultural policy] now days is not nutrition sensitive, so the agriculture people are just contradicting some of the messages [from nutrition]. Sometimes they say 'just produce more and gain more money, not to eat', and sometimes they are just promoting only the saving issue and sometimes they are not just promoting issue related with the consumption of high food and vegetable consumption of dense food for the children especially for the under five children and for the mother. (IDI-13)

These findings resonate with a question raised by (Roberts 2008) as to whether it's a conflict of interest when an agricultural department is "expected to champion and protect both farmers who sell and consumers who buy the same product".

Under GTP-2, the agricultural sector has a range of major targets (table 19, GTP-2) in the areas of production, food security, productivity, trade and marketing and input supply. These may often be complementary to the goals of NNP-2. For example, GTP2 contains targets for improvement in the number of production safety net recipients, the size of the food reserve and in cereal output. It also contains targets around increases in export earnings from major commodities, and these have a complex relationship to nutrition improvement, depending significantly on the pay and conditions of workers in export production (Cramer et al. 2017). In addition, the promotion of exports of food crops, most notably teff, the major staple of Ethiopia and hailed as a new 'superfood', may lead to sharp prices rises on local markets. Despite its success in earning scarce foreign exchange, there have been some criticisms of the partial lifting of export ban on teff, with concern that, however sensitive the policy was to nutrition concerns, it would reduce domestic food security (Secorun 2016; Reda 2015).

- One interviewee explained that there could be difficulties when consensus on the involvement of different governmental ministries could not be reached:

The whole idea of having a national overarching document was there for a long time before that… one of the issues which prevented the launch of even the document was to decide which ministry [should coordinate it], so… they told me that people at parliament and the Prime Minister's Office had to make the final decision. (IDI-17)

Even with the coordinating framework of the GTP and NNP, there can thus be obvious challenges when a policy problem is identified through one sector – in this case based on the indicators of malnutrition and related health – yet must be addressed by action within another sector (e.g. agriculture). There may be differences of opinion on the priority or importance of policy action, clashes in authority between departments who may vie for ownership of policy and interventions, and need for coordination and cooperation that adds additional levels of complication beyond what would be needed in single-sector policymaking (Pelletier et al. 2012; Hoey and Pelletier 2011; Trivedi 2000; Mills 1990). Health sector respondents certainly described that, under NNP-I and GTP-I, nutrition was not sufficiently prioritised in the policy-making of other sectors and that nutrition targets were not sufficiently represented in overarching documents.

These issues suggest questions as to why up-stream nutrition policy-making proved difficult under NNP-I. The interviews also throw light on key issues in the NNP-II, and reinforce the argument that for multi-sectoral policy making, the issue is not only one of aligning interests under GTP-II and NNP-II but also of developing capacity around nutrition in sectors and producing nutrition-relevant evidence. Crucially they suggest that for nutrition to be appropriately framed, the MoA needs to adopt an internal logic that aligns its productivity and trade goals enshrined in GTP-II with NNP-II goals, and devises and monitors policy using nutrition-relevant evidence. More fundamentally, this also requires discussion of trade-offs between multiple and at times competing interests and concerns typical within broader political thinking (Lasswell 1990 [1936]).

IMPLICATIONS FOR 'EVIDENCE INFORMED' NUTRITION POLICY

The challenge of developing and implementing multi-sectoral policy is multifaceted, but interviewees raised two specific challenges in relation to evidence use and policy response. First, although multi-sectoral plans and infrastructure to address malnutrition were in place, the mandate for addressing nutrition lay with the health sector, which was reinforced by the nature of nutrition data collected or used.

Ultimately in terms of evidence use, however, this presents a situation whereby the evidence that has globally (and locally) provided the motivation for action – evidence such as under-five mortality, rates of diarrhoea and infections, prevalence of overweight and obesity – may not have the same importance to many of the key stakeholders required for sustainable, effective, policy action. This is because such evidence may not be judged as relevant by non-health stakeholders if their own institutional logics are based around a different normative position or set of goals. Indeed, respondents reflected on how the framing of relevant evidence could vary between the international discourse and the relevant local institutions cutting across a number of sectors – each with its own idea of what is relevant to justify policy action or inform policy decisions.

Respondents discussed the need for data and research evidence showing impacts on more than just health outcomes (e.g. educational or economic productivity) in order to achieve policy change. One respondent explained:

The impact of malnutrition for example on economic development, you have to quantify it... you have to convert the malnutrition impact in money and the money for the national development. You have to convert the impact of malnutrition for example on education; if a child is malnourished the performance for education will be just... you can tell just like this [...] We get [information on] impact of malnutrition across different sectors. On health, on education on productivity... At every advocacy place we are using those data actually. (IDI-23)

Indeed, as a way of providing multi-sectoral nutrition evidence, the Government of Ethiopia published a report: *The cost of hunger in Ethiopia: Implications for the growth and transformation of Ethiopia*, becoming the first country to engage in the Africa Union's Cost of Hunger exercise (African Union Commission, World Food Programme, and Africa 2012). This report provides economic costing of the long-term impacts of underfive undernutrition, exploring the cost of higher healthcare spending on this group, education costs when these people are in the school system, and the productivity costs as they enter the workforce – and estimates that in 2009, the cost of child undernutrition was 55.5 billion Ethiopian Birr (16.5% of GDP – approximately USD$4.3 billion in Dec 2009).

Ethiopia's early involvement in the cost of hunger exercise demonstrates commitment to the creation of evidence relevant to other sectors. As such, it is a powerful tool to aid multi-sectoral policymaking, and provides evidence relevant to other targets in the GTP-2 plan. However, in itself, it only partially quantifies the goals of NNP-2. While NNP-2 is concerned with the undernutrition of young children, it is also concerned with the undernutrition of adolescents and women. Equally, our health sector respondents described how rising rates of overweight and obesity and their NCD impacts were relevant to nutrition policymaking. So the Cost of Hunger exercise appears only to provide a partial multi-sectoral evidence base.

A final challenge raised in our interviews, however, was the perception that multi-level data from across the country (including decentralised information) was also needed to inform an appropriate nutrition strategy, but that these data were not yet available in sufficient volume. One respondent, for instance, stated:

We are just starting to utilise the available resource at different levels. Information is important for different levels not only central level... I think within the next five years we can get a clear picture of information flow from across different sectors, horizontally as well as vertically. (IDI-23)

These challenges in the evidence base may particularly undermine upstream intervention and planning – for nutrition or other health policy issues. Downie (2016) has described the Government of Ethiopia as particularly outcome oriented, with a centralised drive to achieve 'near term development goals' (pp. vi) While our study was not able to validate this claim, it is worth noting that if a principle focus of the government is for evidence that can show measurable outcomes aligned with core targets on undernutrition, this would presumably incentivise the use of forms of evidence that focus on immediate and direct impacts that can more easily be quantified, such as supplemental nutrition for acute malnutrition cases. The evidence base required for, and useful for, informing the addressing of and evaluating the impact of interventions targeting upstream structural determinants of health including nutrition are much broader, less certain, and often harder to quantify (Bonnefoy et al. 2007; Parkhurst 2017). Accordingly, the intervention types given the greatest attention may be those that are less likely to bring about more systematic and sustained progress over the longer term.

Discussion

The framing of nutrition in Ethiopia is changing, with greater discussion of considering malnutrition in all its forms: undernutrition and micronutrient deficiencies, as well as overweight, obesity and NCDs. Nutrition has also been seen at the highest level of Government as an issue that requires multi-sectoral action. However, our interviews provided a health sector perspective to the problems of target setting and evidence use.

Thus, while there has been a broader framing of nutrition amongst health stakeholders and to some extent in official nutrition policy, overweight- and obesity-related targets are less evident in key documents. While, in theory, responding to nutrition more holistically and multi-sectorally reflects the state of contemporary thinking about the most effective approach to addressing malnutrition, such approaches present particular challenges to the idea of an obvious body of evidence that can simply inform or guide policymaking. One way to understand the limits to this conceptualisation has been to apply an institutional lens, considering the structures in place that influence which evidence is brought to bear on policy decisions and the institutionalised logics that relate to evidence use, which may differ across agencies involved in nutrition policy.

In public health, there is a recognised tension between the need for more structural interventions, and the realities that interventions focussing on treatment or downstream individual approaches can be easier to conceptualise, measure, and evaluate. Even with increased recognition or calls for upstream action, the existing data and evidence may focus policy action on downstream efforts, which appears to remain a challenge for nutrition policy in Ethiopia. Without a solution, this may continue to hamper the implementation of NNP-2.

The more recent 2016 *Situation Analysis of the Nutrition Sector in Ethiopia* document attempts to make agriculture in Ethiopia more nutrition-sensitive through the adoption of dietary diversity as an outcome indicator in the most recent iteration of the Agricultural Growth Program (AGP). It also describes how, for the agricultural sector, appropriate indicators of food security and dietary diversity should be chosen for evaluation of agricultural sector responsibilities (FMoH/UNICEF/EU Situation Analysis of the Nutrition Sector in Ethiopia: 2000–2015 2016). This suggests that while data may block how far dominant ideas may be able to progress in shaping policy, those ideas can work to re-shape which data are generated, potentially providing useful evidence for future approaches to nutrition policy.

An important insight into the challenges faced in evidence use to inform nutrition policy come from March and Olsen's institutional concept of the 'logic of appropriateness', which captures the ways that institutions develop their own internal norms, values, and understandings of how things should work, which are enacted in their operations (March and Olsen 1984, 2011). This idea provides an opportunity for reflection on the unexpected results that can arise when differing logics come into conflict in policy debates.

Different institutional norms, values and logics of appropriateness between the health and agricultural sectors were perceived by the health sector actors in our study (although we acknowledge that greater insight could be obtained by further work interviewing representatives of agriculture and other sectors). Despite the framing given by NNP and GTP, agricultural interests were often considered by our respondents to be driven by productivity targets and associated evaluation, without appropriate inclusion of nutrition objectives. This view resonates with the official acknowledgements of the weaknesses of NNP (above). Respondents also spoke of need for nutrition to be framed in terms of its impact on the country's economic development at times. However, such challenges are not unique to Ethiopia. Balarajan and Reich (2016) have described the challenges posed by different stakeholder narratives of nutrition globally (Balarajan and Reich 2016).

There are many targets that are complementary between sectors, and the *The cost of hunger in Ethiopia: Implications for the growth and transformation of Ethiopia* report helps identify these. In future, the new NNP-2 and GTP-2 may provide a framework to produce rapid progress on those areas where evidence suggests strong mutual gains. An example of such synergy is the fact that one of the initiatives of the NNP-I (2013–2015) was to "*promote and disseminate bio-fortified micronutrient-rich staple food products, such as orange sweet potatoes and quality protein-rich maize.*" This initiative is under the direct influence of the MoA. By allocating necessary attention to this initiative, the MoA not only contributes to the realization of the objectives set forth in the NNP-1, and NNP-2, but also this is a core objective for the MoA itself. Obviously, these areas are particularly likely to advance strongly under the existing multisectoral coordination framework because they talk to evidence and targets that are equally recognised and valued.

Conclusion

This paper has discussed an area of acknowledged weakness in Ethiopia's multi-sectoral nutrition policy framework: that of the role of policymaking with varied, conflicting and missing evidence. It focuses particularly on health stakeholder perspectives, and thus can only explore some of the issues involved. Despite this, it illuminates three issues. First, it helps explain the problems in the coordination of mandates and evidence in NNP-1 and suggests likely areas for continuing challenge under NNP-2. Second, we have argued that there is still a lack of clarity about the role of upstream interventions, and despite a framework for integrating targets through NNP-2 and GTP-2, this may be worsened by the tension with some agricultural sector targets. Here the point is that unified frameworks result from tense, often unseen struggles between conflicting political goals. Third, despite the improvements in the evidence base, we argue that further evidence is needed to inform nutrition policymaking in Ethiopia, and that more evidence is needed to inform policy in non-health sectors on nutrition-specific interventions.

Even though Ethiopia has made progress in terms of nutrition targets and has a strategic framework aiming to address past problems, it shares the challenge of countries elsewhere in addressing nutrition as a multi-sectoral issue. It also provides a useful case of institutional logics and how assumptions about the type and role of policy-relevant evidence for nutrition policy action may not hold across sectors.

Our study takes place at a key moment in nutrition policy making in Ethiopia. Whilst we found that respondents were aware of a variety of nutrition problems and approaches to nutritional issues, our findings contrast with those of Kennedy et al. (2015), who described a 'general consensus' amongst their interview respondents that the 'nutrition problem' in Ethiopia is one of undernutrition (with respondents from a broad range of sectors). This difference may reflect the earlier (2013, rather than at the end of 2014) period of data collection, but may also reflect differences in the methodological and epistemological approach of the two studies. That said, the importance of the focus on undernutrition should not be underestimated. This was also recognised by our respondents as critical and a major challenge, but our research questions particularly endeavoured to probe about other aspects of nutrition policy beyond this dominant frame.

Finally, this paper explored the role that evidence and target-setting can play in informing and influencing the direction of policy development for nutrition. Rather than a simple one-way path from evidence to policy, the case of nutrition has shown the complex interaction of evidence within different conceptualisations of policy problems and responses. These processes play out in a setting where there is a strong steer to unified approaches at the national level. Evidence may not always easily speak to preferred policy responses, and the importance or relevance of different types of evidence may vary across sectors based on varying institutionalised logics by which they purse policy goals. Evidence is not fixed, with new constructions of data and evidence always emerging, and subject to influence by those stakeholders active in the particular policy arena. We thus expect to see continuing evolution of the body of evidence available to inform nutrition policy in Ethiopia, as well as potential changes in how different stakeholders conceptualise the importance of different evidence types.

Acknowledgements We are most grateful to the participation of the study respondents in this research.

This research was conducted as part of the Getting Research into Policy in Health (GRIP-Health) project, supported by a grant from the European Research Council (Project ID#282118).

REFERENCES

African Union Commission, World Food Programme, and United Nations Economic Commission for Africa. 2012. The cost of hunger in Ethiopia: Implications for the growth and transformation of Ethiopia. Addis Ababa.
Balarajan, Y., and M.R. Reich. 2016. Political economy challenges in nutrition. *Globalization and Health* 12: 70.
Benson, T. 2005. *Improving nutrition as a development priority: Addressing undernutrition within national policy processes in sub-Saharan Africa*. Washington, DC: International Food Policy Research Institute.
Bhutta, Z.A., and R.A. Salam. 2012. Global nutrition epidemiology and trends. *Annals of Nutrition & Metabolism* 61 (1): 19.
Bonita, Ruth, Roger Magnusson, Pascal Bovet, Dong Zhao, Deborah C. Malta, Robert Geneau, Il Suh, Kavumpurathu Raman Thankappan, Martin McKee, James Hospedales, Maximilian de Courten, Simon Capewell, and Robert Beaglehole. 2013. Country actions to meet UN commitments on non-communicable diseases: A stepwise approach. *The Lancet* 381 (9866): 575–584. https://doi.org/10.1016/S0140-6736(12)61993-X.
Bonnefoy, J, A. Morgan, M.P. Kelly, J. Butt, and V. Bergman. 2007. Constructing the evidence base on the social determinants of health: A guide. In *Measurement and Evidence Knowledge Network (MEKN)*. Universidad del Desarrollo, Chile, and National Institute for Health and Clinical Excellence, Manchester.
Cramer, C., D. Johnston, C. Oya, and J. Sender. 2017. Fairtrade and labour markets in Ethiopia and Uganda. *Journal of Development Studies* 53 (6): 841–856.
Dangour, A.D., E. Kennedy, and A. Taylor. 2013. Commentary: The changing focus for improving nutrition. *Food and Nutrition Bulletin* 34 (2): 194.
Dorfman, L., and L. Wallack. 2007. Moving nutrition upstream: The case for reframing obesity. *Journal of Nutrition Education and Behavior* 39 (2): S45–S50.
Downie, R. 2016. *Sustaining Improvements to public health in Ethiopia*. A Report of CSIS Global Health Policy Center.
Embassy of the Federal Democratic Republic of Ethiopia. 2016. Disaster Prevention and Preparedness Commission.
Ethiopia Central Statistical Agency and ICF International. 2012. 2011 Ethiopia Demographic and Health Survey: Key findings. Addis Ababa, Ethiopia and Calverton, Maryland, USA: Central Statistical Agency and ICF International.
Ethiopian Academy of Science. 2013. *Report on integration of nutrition into agriculture and health in Ethiopia*. Addis Ababa: Ethiopian Academy of Science.
Federal Democratic Republic of Ethiopia. 1996. National food security strategy. Addis Ababa.
———. 2011. Growth and Transformation Plan (2010/11–2014/15). Addis Ababa.

———. 2016. Growth and Transformation Plan II (GTP II) (2015/16–2019/20). Addis Ababa.

Federal Ministry of Health. 2008. National Nutrition Strategy. http://www.iycn.org/files/National-Nutrition-Strategy.pdf

FMoH/UNICEF/EU Situation Analysis of the Nutrition Sector in Ethiopia: 2000–2015. 2016. Ethiopian Federal Ministry of Health, UNICEF and European Commission Delegation.

Garrett, J., and M. Natalicchio. 2011. Working multisectorially in nutrition: Principles, practices and case studies. IFPRI.

Gillespie, Stuart, Lawrence Haddad, Venkatesh Mannar, Purnima Menon, Nicholas Nisbett, and Maternal, and Child Nutrition Study Group. 2013. The politics of reducing malnutrition: Building commitment and accelerating progress. *The Lancet* 382 (9891): 552–569.

Government of the Federal Democratic Republic of Ethiopia. 2013. National Nutrition Programme: June 2013–June 2015.

———. 2016. National Nutrition Programme II: 2016–2020.

Hazards and Vulnerability Research Institute. 2014. The 1983–1985 Ethiopian Famine. http://webra.cas.sc.edu/hvri/feature/oct2013_dom.aspx

Heaver, R. 2005. *Strengthening country commitment to human development: Lessons from nutrition directions in development series*. Washington, DC: The World Bank.

Hoey, L., and D.L. Pelletier. 2011. The management of conflict in nutrition policy formulation: Choosing growth-monitoring indicators in the context of dual burden. *Food and Nutrition Bulletin* 32 (2 Suppl): S82–S91.

International Food Policy Research Institute. 2015. *Global nutrition report*. Washington, DC: IFPRI.

Kanter, R., H.L. Walls, M. Tak, F. Roberts, and J. Waage. 2015. A conceptual framework for understanding the impacts of agriculture and food system policies on nutrition and health. *Food Security* 7 (4): 767–777.

Kassebaum, N.J. 2014. Global, regional, and national levels and causes of maternal mortality during 1990–2013: A systematic analysis for the Global Burden of Disease Study 2013. *The Lancet* 384 (9947): 980–1004.

Kassie, B.T., H. Hengsdijk, R.P. Rotter, H. Kahiluoto, S. Asseng, and M. van Ittersum. 2013. Adapting to climate variability and change: Experience from cereal-based farming in the Central Rift and Kobo valleys, Ethiopia. *Environment Management* 52 (5): 1115–1131.

Kassie, B.T., R.P. Rotter, H. Hengsdijk, and S. Asseng. 2014. Climate variability and change in the Central Rift Valley of Ethiopia: Challenges for rainfed crop production. *The Journal of Agricultual Science* 152 (1): 58–74.

Keller, E.J. 1992. Drought, war and the politics of famine in Ethiopia and Eritrea. *The Journal of Modern African Studies* 30 (4): 609–624.

Kennedy, E., M. Tessema, T. Hailu, D. Zerfu, A. Belay, G. Ayana, D. Kuche, T. Moges, T. Assefa, A. Samuel, T. Kassaye, H. Fekadu, and J. van Wassenhove. 2015. Multisector nutrition program governance and implementation in Ethiopia: Opportunities and challenges. *Food and Nutrition Policy* 36 (4): S34–S48.

Lachat, Carl, Stephen Otchere, Dominique Roberfroid, Abubakari Abdulai, Florencia Maria Aguirre Seret, Jelena Milesevic, Godfrey Xuereb, Vanessa Candeias, and Patrick Kolsteren. 2013. Diet and physical activity for the prevention of noncommunicable diseases in low-and middle-income countries: A systematic policy review. *PLoS Medicine* 10 (6): e1001465.

Lasswell, H.D. 1990 [1936]. *Politics; who gets what, when, how.* Gloucester: Peter Smith Publisher.

Lowndes, V., and M. Roberts. 2013. *Why institutions matter: The new institutionalism in political science.* Basingstoke: Palgrave Macmillan.

Malik, V.S., W.C. Willet, and F.B. Hu. 2013. Global obesity: Trends, risk factors and policy implications. *National Review of Endocrinology* 9: 13–17.

March, J.G., and J.P. Olsen. 1984. The new institutionalism: Organizational factors in political life. *The American Political Science Review* 78 (3): 734–749.

———. 2011. The logic of appropriateness. In *The Oxford handbook of public policy*, ed. R.E. Goodin, M. Moran, and M. Rein. Oxford: Oxford University Press.

Marmot, M. 2005. Social determinants of health inequalities. *Lancet* 365: 1099–1104.

Mendis, S. 2010. The policy agenda for prevention and control of non-communicable diseases. *British Medical Bulletin* 96: 23–43.

Mills, M.E. 1990. *Conflict resolution and public policy.* New York: Greenwood Press.

Ministry of Health. 2015. Health Sector Transformation Plan (HSTP). The Federal Democratic Republic of Ethiopia, Ministry of Health.

Nabyonga-Orem, J., and R. Mijumbi. 2015. Evidence for informing health policy development in Low-income Countries (LICs): Perspectives of policy actors in Uganda. *International Journal of Health Policy and Management* 4 (5): 285–293.

Nisbett, N., E. Wach, L. Haddad, and S. El Arifeen. 2015. What drives and constrains effective leadership in tackling child undernutrition? Finding from Bangladesh, Ethiopia, India and Kenya. *Food Policy* 53: 33–45.

Nutley, S.M., I. Walter, and H.T.O. Davies. 2007. *Using evidence: how research can inform public services.* Bristol: The Policy Press.

Parkhurst, J.O. 2017. *The politics of evidence: from evidence based policy to the good governance of evidence.* Abingdon: Routledge.

Pelletier, D.L., E.A. Frongillo, S. Gervais, L. Hoey, P. Menon, T. Ngo, R.J. Stoltzfus, A.M. Ahmed, and T. Ahmed. 2012. Nutrition agenda setting, policy formulation and implementation: Lessons from the mainstreaming nutrition initiative. *Health Policy & Planning* 27 (1): 19–31.

Peters, B.G. 2008. Institutional theory: Problems and prospects. In *Debating institutionalism*, ed. B.G. Peters In J. Pierre and G. Stoker, 1–21. Manchester: University of Manchester Press.

Reda, A. 2015. Achieving food security in Ethiopia by promoting productivity of future world food tef: A review. *Advances in Plants & Agriculture Research* 2 (2), 45.

Reinhardt, K., and J. Fanzo. 2014. Addressing chronic malnutrition through multi-sectoral, sustainable approaches: A review of the causes and consequences. *Frontiers in Nutrition* 1: 13.

Roberto, C.A., B. Swinburn, C. Hawkes, T.T.K. Huang, S.A. Costa, M. Ashe, L. Zwicker, J.H. Cawley, and K.D. Brownell. 2015. Patchy progress on obesity prevention: Emerging examples, entrenched barriers, and new thinking. *The Lancet* 385 (9985): 2400–2409.

Roberts, W. 2008. *The no-nonsense guide to world food*. Toronto: New International Publications, Ltd.

Ruel, M.T., H. Alderman, and Maternal and Child Nutrition Study Group. 2013. Nutrition-sensitive interventions and programmes: How can they help to accelerate progress in improving maternal and child nutrition? *The Lancet* 382 (9891): 536–551.

Secorun, L. 2016. Teff could be the next quinoa as Ethiopia boosts exports. https://www.theguardian.com/sustainable-business/2016/oct/14/teff-quinoa-ethiopia-boosts-exports-food-africa

Shiffman, Jeremy. 2006. Donor funding priorities for communicable disease control in the developing world. *Health Policy and Planning* 21 (6): 411–420. https://doi.org/10.1093/heapol/czl028.

Smith, K.E. 2013. *Beyond evidence based policy in public health*. London: Palgrave Macmillan.

Tebekaw, Y., C. Teller, and U. Colon-Ramos. 2014. The burden of underweight and overweight among women in Addis Ababa, Ethiopia. *BMC Public Health* 14: 1126.

Trivedi, P. 2000. How to evaluate performance of government agency: A manual for practitioners. World Bank.

USAID. 2016. Ethiopia. https://www.usaid.gov/ethiopia

Walls, H.L., L. Cornelsen, K. Lock, and R.D. Smith. 2016a. How much priority is given to nutrition and health in the EU Common Agricultural Policy? *Food Policy* 59: 12–23.

Walls, H.L., S. Kadiyala, and R.D. Smith. 2016b. Research and policy for addressing malnutrition in all its forms. *Obesity* 24 (10): 2032.

Webb, P., and J. von Braun. 1994. *Famine and food security in Ethiopia: Lessons for Africa*. Chichester: Wiley.
Weiss, C.H. 1979. The many meanings of research utilization. *Public Administration Review* 39 (5): 426–431.
WHO. 2013. *Global nutrition policy review: What does it take to scale up nutrition action?* Geneva: World Health Organization.
World Bank. 2013. *Improving nutrition through multisectoral approaches*. Washington, DC: World Bank.
World Food Programme. 2017. Productive Safety Net Programme in Ethiopia. https://www.wfp.org/content/protective-safety-net-programme-ethiopia
Zello, G.A. 2015. Natinal nutrtion programs in emering countries: Coping with the double burden of malnutrition and obesity in Ethiopia. *Canadian Journal of Diabetes* 39: S4.

Open Access This chapter is licensed under the terms of the Creative Commons Attribution 4.0 International License (http://creativecommons.org/licenses/by/4.0/), which permits use, sharing, adaptation, distribution and reproduction in any medium or format, as long as you give appropriate credit to the original author(s) and the source, provide a link to the Creative Commons license and indicate if changes were made.

The images or other third party material in this chapter are included in the chapter's Creative Commons license, unless indicated otherwise in a credit line to the material. If material is not included in the chapter's Creative Commons license and your intended use is not permitted by statutory regulation or exceeds the permitted use, you will need to obtain permission directly from the copyright holder.

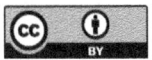

CHAPTER 4

The Use of Evidence in Health Policy in Ghana: Implications for Accountability and Democratic Governance

Elisa Vecchione and Justin Parkhurst

INTRODUCTION

This chapter explores some of the governmental implications of particular uses of policy relevant data and evidence for health policymaking in Ghana. In particular it looks beyond issues of technical capacity to include issues of political responsibility—namely responsibility to use evidence, to take it into account, and to account for it. It is worth noting that claims that

---

This chapter presents an edited version of a paper first published as:
Vecchione, E., and J. Parkhurst (2015). The use of evidence within policy evaluation in health in Ghana: Implications for accountability and democratic governance. *European Policy Analysis* 1 (2): 111–131.

E. Vecchione (✉)
London School of Hygiene and Tropical Medicine, London, UK
e-mail: e.vecchione@ucl.ac.uk

J. Parkhurst
London School of Economics and Political Science, London, UK
e-mail: j.parkhurst@lse.ac.uk

© The Author(s) 2018
J. Parkhurst et al. (eds.), *Evidence Use in Health Policy Making*, International Series on Public Policy,
https://doi.org/10.1007/978-3-319-93467-9_4

evidence can improve accountability practices and democratic decisions are seen within some current calls for 'evidence-based policymaking' (EBPM) (c.f: Weisburd and Neyroud 2011; Clarence 2002), but the way such improvement should occur remains vague and under-investigated. From a general decision-making perspective, the use of evidence serves to inform decisions and to make them more 'rational'. In addition, explicit use of evidence potentially improves transparency and along with it the accountability of decisions. However, accountability is not an inherent property of decisions. It is a practice put into being by policy agents and procedures.

This chapter uses a case study of Ghana in order to explore how uses of evidence for national planning link with concepts of accountability, and what political effects particular uses of evidence can produce. The analysis focuses on a specific stage of the policy cycle, namely the evaluation process of health policies and programs. Policy evaluation has indeed been assigned an ever important role in policymaking through the idea that decisions are 'better' when they can be *tested* (Weiss 1999). Under this view, policy evaluation combines governance needs for more efficient policy outcomes with legitimacy quests for more democratic decision processes and outcomes. Evidence plays a prominent role in enabling such tests and validating decisions according to their outcomes. Indeed, the mechanisms by which evidence from evaluation systems work to inform future policy choices can be seen as a process by which technical measurements of policy achievements take on political value in shaping policy directions. But questions remain about how such translation occurs in practice; and how it connects concepts of efficient and legitimate policymaking. These are important questions which can be obscured by the apolitical calls for 'evidence use' in policymaking. In this chapter, the term 'evaluation' principally refers to data related to performance monitoring, but also refers to how such data are used to evaluate policy choices as well.

As a parliamentary democracy and an aid-recipient country,[1] Ghana provides an interesting arena in which to investigate the democratic implications of evidence use in policymaking, namely by applying the concerns, which have traditionally been applied to more high-income countries, over the expansion of expert-based decision-making structures outside

---

[1] A recent estimate from the U.S. Global Health Initiative in Ghana shows that 40% of the national budget comes from development assistance (available at http://www.ghi.gov/wherewework/docs/ghanastrategy.pdf).

national polities (Barnett and Finnemore 1999) and the consequent balance between governance improvements and legitimacy decisions.

In order to investigate the practical applications of evidence use in policy evaluation in Ghana, and its links to accountability, this paper combines theoretical and empirical considerations as follows: First, we briefly review theoretical arguments drawn from public administration and policy studies to understand how the concepts of accountability and evidence use have been associated in governance and policymaking studies. We then investigate such association through empirical analysis of health policy in Ghana. Finally, we discuss the theoretical contributions in light of both our empirical findings and sociological approaches to policymaking.

Our empirical analysis is principally informed by a set of 24 in-depth interviews following a semi-structured approach, conducted in 2014 with a set of stakeholders in Ghanaian health policy—including representatives of the Ministry of Health (MoH), the Ghana Health Service (GHS), international development partners (DP), local nongovernment organizations (LNGOs), and members of parliament (MP). When specific interviewees are cited in this paper, they are designated by an anonymous number and one of these acronyms. The interviews aimed to understand the institutional role and position of each interviewee with respect to other actors in the health sector, as well as their perception and understanding of evidence use in health policymaking. Data analysis partly benefitted from the use of qualitative tools, such coding using the Nvivo qualitative software package, and from the triangulation with other sources of data including official documents.

Evaluation and Accountability Within a Policy Space

In its simplest form, accountability links the capacity to *evaluate* decision outcomes to the idea of *controlling* political agency (Dubnick and Frederickson 2011). As per the principal-agent model, the *elected* principal confers the *delegated* administrative 'agent' the power to apply directives, while endowing the agent with a margin of discretion. Hence, the need to oversee her decisions by making the agent accountable for them (Pratt and Zeckhauser 1991). In principle, evidence helps operationalize accountability rules: by informing decisions within the range of discretion that authorities have over decisions, and by defining the legitimacy of decisions.

Under this conceptualization of accountability and evidence use, the process of evaluating decisions becomes more than a simple managerial or technical function. Rather, evaluation evidence serves as a powerful tool for testing the achievement of policy objectives, directing policy discussions, validating a particular policy strategy, and rewarding it by allocating more funds or prolonging its life cycle. However, the contribution of evidence to accountability depends on the extent to which evidence also exposes decisions to judgment and contestation (Heidelberg 2015).

Precisely for these reasons of multiple functionality of evidence use, it is critical to analyze how pieces of evidence shift from being used for simple technical measurement, to more normative judging (*valuation*) of policy. Applying an institutional lens, however, means that we are particularly interested in how this shift can often occur within a specific policy space created by formalized evaluation processes. These insights provide a framework in which we can analyze how the policy evaluation process provides space for participation and contestation among stakeholders over the use of evidence to judge policy value. It further allows reflection on how rules of accountability within those evaluation processes serve to establish power relations and set the spaces through which such contestation takes place.

Evidence and Health Sector Assessment in Ghana

Ghana is a lower-middle income country located in Western Africa. It is often considered one of the more democratic and developed of Sub-Saharan African nations, but it still suffers from significant resource limitations. The structure of the health system in Ghana follows the basics of functional separation between decision making and implementation in policymaking (Cassels 1995). Due to concerns over efficiency, some functions traditionally concentrated in the MoH were delegated to technical agencies benefitting from a certain degree of independence from government and discretion. The GHS is an autonomous Executive Agency of the MoH and represents one of the most important policy implementation bodies in the health sector, responsible for managing and operating all public health facilities and tasked with planning, implementation, monitoring and performance assessment of health programmes and services (Adjei 2003). The GHS has considerable power in the health sector. It was set upon the managerial objective of improving service delivery in Ghana, namely by deconcentrating the vertical structure of programs under the

MoH (e.g., HIV, TBA, etc.) into local units of management and implementation (Cassels and Janovsky 1992). In practice, however, the GHS provides a parallel structure of hierarchical governance (Cassels and Janovsky 1992) serving the broader political objective of bringing coherence into the health system.

The Health Information Management Department (HIMD) of the Policy, Planning, Monitoring, and Evaluation (PPME) division was established within the GHS as the focal unit responsible for the collection, analysis, reporting, and presentation of health service information (Adjei 2003). Regional and the District level offices were established with each having their own Health Administrations (RHAs and DHAs) and each should report to the higher hierarchical level (Adjei 2003) (see Fig. 4.1) (Couttolenc 2012). In spite of some problems—e.g. overlapping responsibilities at times emerging across managerial units and local political authorities (Couttolenc 2012),[2] a fairly well formalized structure of accountability exists (within the GHS and between the GHS and the MoH), integrated with a systematic practice of reporting and reviewing performances of implementation policies, as widely acknowledged by our interviewees at the GHS.

The connection between evidence use and accountability in the Ghana health system can be seen in the integration of the Health Information Management Department (HIMD) within this national system of accountability. The HIMD's specific task is to gather health information such as administrative, demographic, and clinical data—typically collected through desk review, although sometimes accompanied by interviews (Zakariah 2014). This is fed upwards from facility to district to region and, ultimately, to central health management levels in order to inform health sector performances (for more details see Ghana Health Service 2012, p. 30). The Centre for Health Information Management within the HIMD collects the data from the district level through the software called the District Health Information Management Information System, and then sends it to the regional level. The aim of this procedure is to collect information

---

[2] Confusion and overlapping responsibilities are mainly due to the fact that the deconcentration of health services as under the Ghana Health Service and Teaching Hospitals Act 525 of 1996, has not yet produced full delegation of power to the local assemblies representing the political authority at the district level as in the Local Government Act 462 of 1993 (Couttolenc 2012). For instance, one local key informant explained that, as consequence of incomplete decentralization, there exists a dual hierarchy in the lines of accountability of the DHA, which has to report back to both the district assembly and to the regional director.

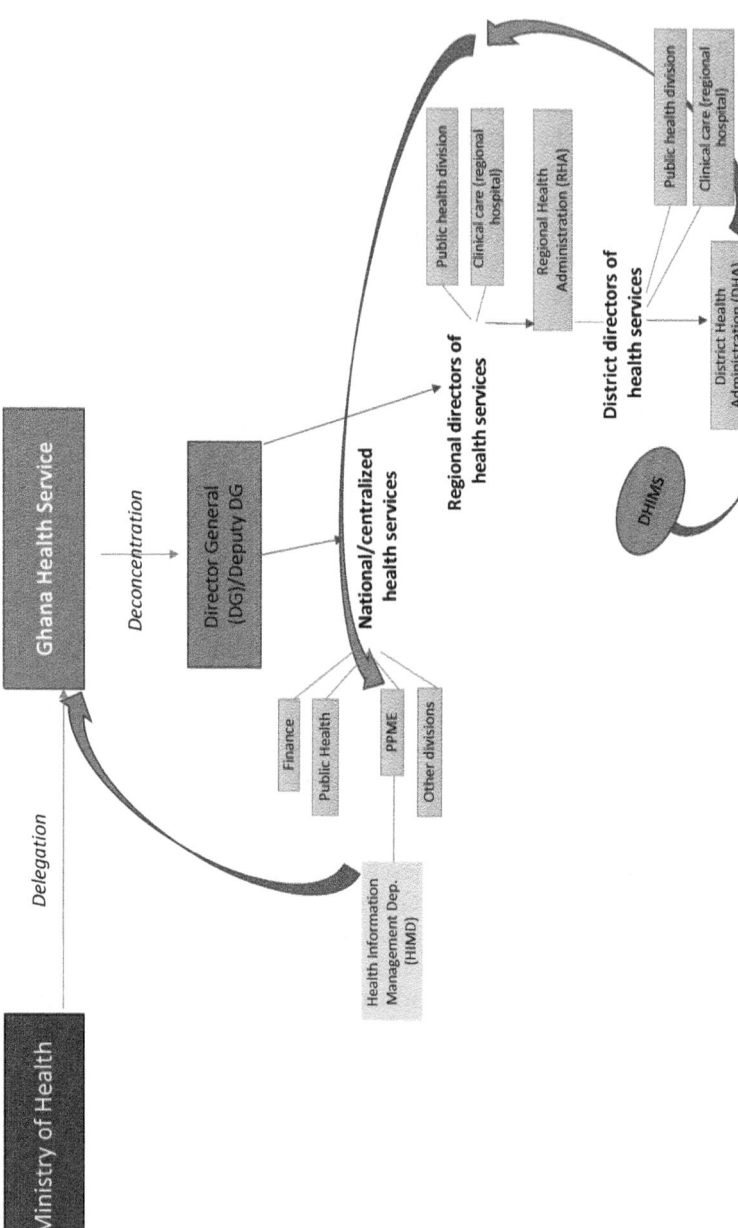

Fig. 4.1 The governance structure of health policy in Ghana. (Adapted from Adjei 2003, regional district administration, GHS, http://www.ghanahealthservice.org/ghs-subcategory.php?cid=&scid=44 Others: http://solutionscenter.nethope.org/case_studies/view/district-health-information-management-system-dhims-ii-the-data-challenge-f)

from the district up to the national level in order to support each Ministerial Agency within the health sector—not only the GHS—with the implementation of their respective strategies established in their 'Programmes of Work' (POWs). Each Agency assesses its progress in implementing the POWs through an in-house Monitoring & Evaluation (M&E) plan, which relies on the information produced by the HIMD. The results of M&E outcomes should finally converge each year into the Interagency/Health Sector Performance Review.

Therefore, a combined mechanism of information diffusion and evaluation of performance exists in Ghana that ties the health governance structure into a system based on a structured review process: operating internally at each administrative level and vertically between district, regional, and headquarter managers via peer-review meetings.

ACCOUNTABILITY, EVALUATION AND POWER IN GHANAIAN HEALTH POLICY

In addition to the process described above combining information and evaluation within the Ghanaian hierarchy, a 'Holistic Assessment tool' has been developed to guide interagency performance review. The Holistic Assessment tool was established within the framework of the Common Management Arrangement (CMA), which governs and set the rules for partnership between the MoH and international donors.

As we will discuss, the tool functions as interface between the MoH, responsible for the health sector performance, and international donor agencies, which demand accountability of performances to the MoH.

The CMA was conceived to address the problem of parallel donor systems and increased aid transaction costs. Now in its third iteration (CMA III), the CMA itself was originally introduced in 1997 with the national health sector reform of decentralizing service delivery—the creation of the GHS being one of the main outcomes—under the sponsorship of the World Health Organization (Ghana Health Sector 2012, p. 5). A health-sector-wide approach was established along with a pooled funding account of donor funds managed by the MoH (Pallas et al. 2015). The method to govern this new framework of collaboration was the Holistic Assessment (IHP+ 2003).

The use of sector-wide indicators, milestones, and targets are a key component of the Holistic Assessment tool. These are established at the national level within the four-year Health Sector Medium Term Development Plan (HSMTDP) and are (re-)formulated each year with the programme of work (POW) that the MoH prepares in line with the objectives of the national health strategy as set in the HSMTDP.[3] Milestones, targets, and indicators at the local level are derived from national equivalents. The data generated by the HIMD from the district to the national level are devoted to fill sector-wide indicators specified in the HSMTDP from which health sector agencies draw their own POWs and implementation strategies (Nyonator et al. 2014). Targets, are negotiated between the GHS and relevant decentralized bodies to administer DPs' funds across the national, regional and district level.[4]

The Holistic Assessment tool is also used by international partners to assess health sector performances. Thus, international donors are involved in the process of selecting indicators, targets and milestones. Information appears to indicate that performance indicators get established and revised each November of the year during the Business Meeting between the MoH and DP (Ghana Health Sector 2012).[5] Based on these indicators, the Holistic Assessment reports a score for each health sector objective established within the annual POW, e.g., bridging equity gaps in health care, improving efficiency, and effectiveness in the health system. A score of +1 is attributed if the indicator has attained the set target, 0 if it just show a good trend, −1 if the target has been missed (IHP+ 2003, pp. 37–38).

Interviews conducted with both administrative officials of the MoH and DP confirmed that, besides the senior managers meeting at the GHS, the main venue for research dissemination and discussion of evidence was

---

[3] The HSMTDP is prepared by the MoH and its Ministries, Departments, and Agencies under the guidance of the National Development Commission and sets the objectives of the national health strategy over a period of four years.

[4] There are several Budget and Management Centres spread throughout the three administrative and facility levels. The headquarters of the GHS is managed as one of them; 10 Regional Health Administration, 8 Regional Hospitals, 110 District Health Administrations, and 95 District Hospitals (GHS, available at http://www.ghanahealthservice.org/ghs-sub-category.php?cid=&scid=43).

[5] There are three business meetings. The business meeting during the April health summit will assess the sector Performance Assessment Framework (PAF) to feed into the Multi-Donor Budget Support dialogue. The second business meeting in August will review the sector's progress from the beginning of the year to date and provide an opportunity to table new issues. The business meeting in November will be devoted to planning and budgeting. The meeting will discuss and agree on health sector plans and associated budget for the ensuing year. It will also agree on indicators for the PAF based on the sector program that was presented and discussed. Finally, and "Aide Memoire" will be signed by the Ministry of Health and representatives of Development Partners that records the decisions taken during the business meeting of November.

the Health Summit—the annual meeting in which DP and government discussed the Holistic Assessment of the health sector (Interviews MoH-1, DP-1, DP-2, DP-3). Indeed, according to one MoH official, the Health Summit is "the key policymaking structure within the sector" (MoH-1). The presentation of the Holistic Assessment to the Health Summit is to provide the mechanism for all sector partners to review performance and assess the level of compliance with the CMA. However, this mechanism of data utilisation serves another purpose besides coordination between different levels of health system governance: it makes the system evaluable by external reviewers. However, the CMA clearly states that the use of the Holistic Assessment tool should be made "in line with the principles of *mutual accountability*" between the MoH and the donors (Ghana Health Sector 2012, p. 7—emphasis added) showing that the Health Summit represents not only an additional venue of evaluation, but also an additional system of accountability in which the MoH is accountable to DP for the overall performance of the health sector.

The Accountability Implications of Uses of Evidence

The creation of a second system of accountability external and parallel to the hierarchical structure of management of the Ghana health system could in theory be managed through the use of common tools for evaluation, which might ensure the alignment and coordination between the two systems of accountability (and evaluation). However, the scores attributed to each target in the Holistic Assessment entails some political judgment of success and failure, raising questions of responsibility and authority to decide on these outcomes (Bovens et al. 2006). Having two accountability systems driven by different stakeholders thus can make it unclear to whom responsibility and liability issues should be referred.

The World Health Organizatoin's description of Ministries of Health as having key 'stewardship' roles in country health decision making (World Health Organization 2000) could imply that the MoH is responsible for the health sector performance and should have overarching authority over relevant stakeholders, active in the health sector including NGOs, international donors, health agencies, academics, health associations, etc. In practice this is not the case, as each stakeholder has its own power to influence the outcome of policy evaluation and, accordingly, influence or bypass accountability structures in place. The ability to do this, in turn, depends on the capacity of each stakeholder to use evidence as a tool for applying its scrutiny to policy performances and defining its discretion in guiding future policy directions; hence, evidence appears as a powerful tool for stakeholders to negotiate their own position with respect to the other participants.

Technical Evaluation and Accountability Mechanisms

Indicators aim to 'indicate' (rather than prove) whether some programmatic situation is still relevant to be considered within a certain policy perspective or whether new situations have emerged that affect policy trajectories. As in the case of Ghana, the HIMD has primarily the duty to 'fill'—rather than create—indicators, as indicators are generally established by international bodies such as the WHO; however, our interviews stated that some margin of discretion over data selection always exists, especially when data are lacking. Also, discretion exists in the very use of indicators to produce reports and draw political attention. So, for instance, one interviewee indicated that the Director General of the GHS can request specific data or indicators that do not fall into the HSTMDP (GHS-1). The discretion over data and indicators could also be seen in the way that particular pieces of data, or particular results of analysis, are promoted by bureaucrats within the HIMD to influence policymakers (GHS-1).

The discretion in filling indicators with data is not a problem per se, neither is selecting specific indicators to promote political awareness over certain issues; on the contrary, discretion is a typical characteristic of technical agencies supposed to simplify very complex situations and enhance the quality and pace of policy decisions. However, discretion raises questions if it is exclusively driven by bureaucracy, in the absence of political engagement to use information in a way that reflects political priorities. As a general consideration, this is a technical problem of managerial accountability relationships: in a typical principal-agent perspective, the 'principal' should guide the 'agent' in the implementation of policy objectives (Pratt and Zeckhauser 1991). In the case of Ghana, an additional concern relates to the fact that the production of indicators and the political values built into them will be used as a policy tool for negotiation (i.e., the Holistic Assessment tool) during the Health Summit. The holistic assessment of progress is indeed meant to be *presented* and *discussed* during the Health Summit and *negotiated* and *agreed* upon by the MoH and Partners at the immediately subsequent business meeting in April (Ghana Health Sector 2012, p. 20). Indeed, the outcome of the health sector assessment serves as the basis for discussing the Performance Assessment Framework (PAF) for Multi-Donor Budget Support during the business meeting following the Health Summit (Ghana Health Sector 2012).[6] Therefore, the CMA sets the framework for both constructing evidence—by specifying how the Holistic Assessment tool should be used—and deciding which evidence should be taken as relevant for future planning.

The case of Ghana shows that the use of evidence does not respond to a purely *informative* concern of enhancing the quality of decisions and anticipating the consequences of actions; it also responds to the need to *justify* decisions at the moment of the Health Summit, hence to negotiate the value of the actions that may follow (Boltanski and Thévenot 2006). Further, the power of DP to influence the selection and evaluation of indicators influences the outcome of the negotiating process and the setting of future policy directions. Indeed, the capacity that stakeholders have to influence each other's views often reflects an adversarial process, in which the construction of policy meaning occurs through negotiation between competing views over policy performances and the subsequent judgments on future policy directions (Bovens et al. 2006). Evidence can be used to arbitrate such adversarial process, but at the same time, where disparity emerges as to the capacity to employ it, evidence can end up determining policy directions.

Excluding coercion, the power that each actor has to influence the process in which policy value get shaped partly rests in the way accountability structures establish common rules for participation and value discussions. These rules, in turn, get operationalized by stakeholders through the selection, activation, and evaluation of policy evaluation tools (Pearce et al. 2014). And indeed these tools create the conditions for setting different types of public spaces of discussion while realistically admitting only those participants with the capacity to provide insights and feedback. For instance, one of our interviewees from the MoH complained about the superior technical capacity of DP to produce evidence of performances (GHS-1). This asymmetry is problematic in two respects: on the one hand, Ghanaian officials have little capacity to enter the technical discussion, hence to raise issues of political relevance connected to them, due to a lack of counteracting arguments.

[6] See *supra* note 6.

On the other hand, the absence of clear problem setting and policy directions established by the MoH makes the discussion dominated by technical considerations of policy implementation performance. Interviewees from both DP and NGOs (DP-3 and LNGO-1) recognized such absence as problematic. In the wording of one representative of an international agency (DP-3), health policy in Ghana is only conceived in operational and strategic terms by the government and never in terms of policy objectives; accordingly, indicators are set only in the form of outcomes (e.g., how many new hospitals have been built?) rather than impacts (e.g., how much child mortality has diminished?). On a different level, an NGO representative (LNGO-1) explained that the Ghana Coalition of NGOs in Health (http://www.ghanahealthngos.net/) has recently decided to challenge the government on health priorities by creating a concurrent space of advocacy and evidence use; the objective being to produce an alternative evidence-based report and submit it to the parliament select committee on health in order to influence health financing. However, it has been reported that the Parliament has very little power in influencing actual health policy outcomes (Ayee 2002) as some of our interviewees confirmed. It was explained, for instance, that the Parliament lacks the financial resources to /commission its own inquiries and studies, which could allow it to have greater say in the direction of health policy. This makes Parliament's influence over domestic policy dependent on external aid provided directly to the legislature, for instance for organizing meetings with the civil society (DP-3, MEP-1 DP-1); at the same time, such dependence renders the Parliament practically impotent to have a say in the approval of sectoral budgets (Ayee 2002).

Therefore, evidence use in this policy space centres mainly on the use of common indicators, which might fail to link evaluation to 'accountable' (and potentially more democratic) decisions. The reason draws precisely on the duality of both evidence use and accountability relationships. In the first case, evidence use is both an informative and justificatory policy tool; in the second, accountability relationships envisage at the same time reporting on performances and policy achievements, and exposing performances to some judgments and deliberation.

Evidence Use and Policy Value Judgements

As much as a practical investigation on the use of evidence in policy evaluation has revealed the existence of structures of power, it has also revealed that policy evaluation is not only a technical process of assessment, but a political process of value formation and judgment. In the case of Ghana, the health policymaking process sees the two typical phases of policy evaluation: (i) evidence synthesis and (ii) learning (i.e. evaluation and valuation), disjointed into two separate spaces of accountability. One is structured around a decentralized structure of governance, whereas the other relies on the partnership between donors and the MoH. Whereas the use of evidence—inscribed in the Holistic Assessment tool—is in principle envisaged in bringing these two spaces together, they remain separated. This situation demonstrated that the relation between technical evaluation and political accountability is not always linear, nor can it be fixed by calls for more evidence use. Instead, looking at the systems of accountability in place along with the practices inscribed into them is crucial to understand the democratic implications of evidence use. In conducting policy evaluation, accountability relationships are important in that they help to set, or reconfigure, the power and influence between stakeholders and decision makers. Accountability is a quite elusive but powerful concept that, broadly speaking, indicates the range of responsiveness of policymakers to stakeholders' interests and values. During— and in contribution to—policy evaluation, interests and ideas of stakeholders become actionable through the way policy outcomes are assessed and policy directions are then selected or altered.

Further, by making political values exposed to public judgment and contestation (Heidelberg 2015), accountability goes beyond simplistic checks of stakeholders' interests and enables a process of continuous reconstruction of political values. In this sense, accountability structures are important not only to shape authority relationships, but also to activate a social mechanism of participation in which the principles of an ideal relationship between those who govern and those who are governed (Bovens 2010; Flinders 2011; Heidelberg 2015; Koppell 2005; Salminen and Lehto 2012) are continuously recreated each time they are 'tested' against legitimacy considerations (Rosanvallon 2011). In turn, the capacity to use knowledge and evidence becomes crucial to (re-)organize such principles through mechanisms of responsiveness and degrees of scrutiny over policymakers' decisions; hence, crucial to operationalize accountability.

Conclusions

In this chapter, we have explored the implications of the use of evidence for democratic decision making by looking at the accountability structures in Ghana. The Health Summit in Ghana revealed the importance of the policy evaluation stage within the policymaking process for understanding the effects of the use of evidence in policymaking—in terms of how the use of data goes beyond technical measurement, and serves to establish political judgements and affect policy choices. In this process, we found that use of evidence is a means through which power is exercised. Also, the use policy evaluation within the Health Summit reveals the role of evidence use in both informing and justifying decisions and its relevance for understanding how accountability relationships matter in structuring power relations. The structure of the accountability relationship, therefore, provides the basis for discussing issues of democratic decision making connected to the use of evidence in policymaking. Indeed, the involvement of international donors, responsible for funding a significant amount of health services, can challenge national structures of authority and accountability that exist within the existing governance structure of the state.

International donors often champion the language of evidence based policymaking, while simultaneously embracing the language of good governance and democratic representation in aid-recipient countries. As the case of Ghana has showed, however, it is important that donors involved in processes of evidence use to inform policy—either by extracting local data to generate their own assessments or in constructing indicators to serve as evaluation tools—consciously consider the potential implications these practices have over local accountability mechanisms along with possible legitimacy concerns. Data created to evaluate (or monitor the performance of) a health sector's functioning may often be described as purely technical tools. Yet when such data are used to inform policy and planning, they can have direct political implications, reflecting the political realities of decision making and planning structures in a country. As shown here, their use can create new accountability systems and thus raise questions over governance and influence over local policy decisions.

References

Adjei, Emmanuel. 2003. Health sector reforms and health information in Ghana. *Information Development* 19 (4): 256–264. https://doi.org/10.1177/026666690301900405.

Ayee, Joseph. 2002. Governance, institutional reforms, and policy outcomes in Ghana. In *Better governance and public policy. Capacity building and democratic renewal in Africa*, ed. Dele Olowu and Soumana Sako, 173–191. Bloomfield: Kumarian Press.

Barnett, Michael N., and Martha Finnemore. 1999. The politics, power, and pathologies of international organizations. *International Organization* 53 (4): 699–732. https://doi.org/10.1162/002081899551048.

Boltanski, Luc, and Laurent Thévenot. 2006. *On Justification: Economies of worth*. Princeton: Princeton University Press.

Bovens, Mark. 2010. Two concepts of accountability: Accountability as a virtue and as a mechanism. *West European Politics* 33 (5): 946–967. https://doi.org/10.1080/01402382.2010.486119.

Bovens, Mark, Paul't Hart, and Sanneke Kuipers. 2006. The politics of policy evaluation. In *The Oxford handbook of public policy*, ed. Michael Moran, Martin Rein, and Robert E. Goodin, 319–335. Oxford: Oxford University Press.

Cassels, Andrew. 1995. Health sector reform: Key issues in less developed countries. *Journal of International Development* 7 (3): 329–347. https://doi.org/10.1002/jid.3380070303.

Cassels, Andrew, and Katja Janovsky. 1992. A time of change: Health policy, planning and organization in Ghana. *Health Policy and Planning* 7 (2): 144–154.

Clarence, Emma. 2002. Technocracy reinvented: The new evidence based policy movement. *Public Policy and Administration* 17 (3): 1–11.

Couttolenc, Bernard F. 2012. *Decentralization and governance in the Ghana Health Sector, World Bank Studies*: The World Bank. https://doi.org/10.1596/978-0-8213-9589-9.

Dubnick, Melvin, and George H. Frederickson. 2011. *Public accountability: Performance measurement, the extended state, and the search for trust*. Washington, DC: National Academy of Public Administration.

Flinders, Matthew. 2011. Daring to be a Daniel: The pathology of politicized accountability in a monitory democracy. *Administration & Society* 43 (5): 595–619. https://doi.org/10.1177/0095399711403899.

Ghana Health Sector. 2012. Common management arrangements for implementation of the sector medium-term development plan. Revised Draft. Ghana Health Service.

Heidelberg, Roy L. 2015. Political accountability and spaces of contestation. *Administration & Society* 0095399715581033. https://doi.org/10.1177/0095399715581033.

IHP+. 2003. *Joint annual health sector reviews: A review of experience*. Produced for IHP+ by HERA (Belgium). Available at: https://www.uhc2030.org/fileadmin/uploads/ihp/Documents/Upcoming_events/JAR%20Final%20Report%20Feb2013.pdf.

Koppell, Jonathan G.S. 2005. Pathologies of accountability: ICANN and the challenge of "multiple accountabilities disorder". *Public Administration Review* 65 (1): 94–108. https://doi.org/10.1111/j.1540-6210.2005.00434.x.

Nyonator, Frank, Anthony Ofosu, Mabel Segbafah, and Selassi d'Almeida. 2014. Monitoring and evaluating progress towards universal health coverage in Ghana. *PLoS Medicine* 11 (9): e1001691.

Pallas, Sarah Wood, Justice Nonvignon, Moses Aikins, and Jennifer Prah. 2015. Responses to donor proliferation in Ghana's health sector: A qualitative case study. *Bulletin of the World Health Organisation* 93: 11–18.
Pearce, Warren, Anna Wesselink, and Hal Colebatch. 2014. Evidence and meaning in policy making. *Evidence & Policy: A Journal of Research, Debate and Practice* 10 (2): 161–165.
Pratt, John W., and Richard Zeckhauser. 1991. Principals and agents: An overview. In *Principals and agents: The structure of business*, ed. John W. Pratt and Richard Zeckhauser. Boston: Harvard Business School Press.
Rosanvallon, Pierre. 2011. *Democratic legitimacy: Impartiality, reflexivity, proximity*. Woodstock: Princeton University Press.
Salminen, Ari, and Kirsi Lehto. 2012. Accountable to whom? Exploring the challenge of multiple accountabilities in finnish public administration. *Halduskultuur – Administrative Culture* 13 (2): 147–162.
Weisburd, David, and Peter Neyroud. 2011. New perspectives on policing. Harvard Kennedy School, Program in Criminal Justice Policy and Management.
Weiss, Carol. H. (1999). The Interface between *Evaluation* and Public Policy. *Evaluation* 5 (4): 468–486. https://doi.org/10.1177/135638909900500408.
World Health Organization. 2000. *The world health report 2000, health systems: Improving performance*. Geneva: The World Health Organization.
Zakariah, Afisah. 2014. Holistic assessment of the health sector performance for 2013. 2014 April Health Summit, GIMPA University, Accra.

Open Access This chapter is licensed under the terms of the Creative Commons Attribution 4.0 International License (http://creativecommons.org/licenses/by/4.0/), which permits use, sharing, adaptation, distribution and reproduction in any medium or format, as long as you give appropriate credit to the original author(s) and the source, provide a link to the Creative Commons license and indicate if changes were made.

The images or other third party material in this chapter are included in the chapter's Creative Commons license, unless indicated otherwise in a credit line to the material. If material is not included in the chapter's Creative Commons license and your intended use is not permitted by statutory regulation or exceeds the permitted use, you will need to obtain permission directly from the copyright holder.

CHAPTER 5

Using Evidence in a Highly Fragmented Legislature: The Case of Colombia's Health System Reform

Arturo Alvarez-Rosete and Benjamin Hawkins

INTRODUCTION

This chapter examines how evidence is used in major policy health policy initiatives in a highly contested political context. Through a case study of legislation proposed in the context of Colombia's ongoing health systems reformed process, it explores how such use is affected by the specific role played by the legislature within a highly fragmented polity. We use an institutionalist framework to identify three concentric layers of fragmentation: at the social, political and administrative levels. The former refers to macro levels social structures and factors shaping Colombian society and politics, including the ongoing armed conflict as associated social cleavages which have loomed over Colombian society for decades. At the second level, Colombian politics is characterised by deep divisions and political cleavages along party lines, coupled with weak party structures. This results in a highly fluid political terrain in which new parties may

A. Alvarez-Rosete (✉) • B. Hawkins
London School of Hygiene and Tropical Medicine, London, UK
e-mail: arturo.alvarez-rosete@lshtm.ac.uk; ben.hawkins@lshtm.ac.uk

© The Author(s) 2018
J. Parkhurst et al. (eds.), *Evidence Use in Health Policy Making*,
International Series on Public Policy,
https://doi.org/10.1007/978-3-319-93467-9_5

quickly emerge and disintegrate, and are often held together by 'political strongmen' around which actors coalesce. At the administrative level, the weakness of the legislative and executive branches and corruption endemic in Colombian politics lead to further fragmentation and inefficiency in decision making with the judiciary stepping into the power vacuum to address the most pressing health systems issues (Hawkins and Alvarez Rosete 2017).

The role of the Colombian legislature in the health policy process has to be understood against this challenging backdrop of its recent political and societal history. In the last decade, Colombia's democracy began the long and difficult process of addressing and moving beyond deeply embedded political and societal conflicts in the form of terrorism, internal armed conflict, the illicit drug trade, clientelism and political corruption, which collectively led to the "partial collapse" of the state in the late 1980s (Bejarano and Pizarro 2002). This was reflected in Colombia's low ranking in the World Bank's Worldwide Governance Indicators (WGIs) project on "Political Stability and Absence of Violence/Terrorism", "Rule of Law" and "Voice and Accountability".[1] However, in September 2016, the World Bank president Jim Yong Kim welcomed advances in the peace process aimed at ending the internal armed conflicts, stating that "the country is closer than ever to putting an end to this vicious cycle, and to starting the long and challenging process of transformation and territorial development" (Kim 2016).

[1] The Worldwide Governance Indicators project reports aggregate and individual governance indicators for over 200 countries over the period 1996–2015, for six dimensions of governance: Voice and Accountability; Political Stability and Absence of Violence/Terrorism; Government Effectiveness; Regulatory Quality; Rule of Law; and Control of Corruption.

"Political Stability and Absence of Violence/Terrorism" captures perceptions of the likelihood that the government will be destabilized or overthrown by unconstitutional or violent means, including politically-motivated violence and terrorism. In this dimension, Colombia scored a percentile rank of: 8.2 (1996), 0.97 (2003), 12.3 (2011) and 12.38 (2015).

"Rule of Law" captures perceptions of the extent to which agents have confidence in and abide by the rules of society, and in particular the quality of contract enforcement, property rights, the police, and the courts, as well as the likelihood of crime and violence. In this dimension, Colombia scored a percentile rank of: 22.01 (1996), 26.32 (2003), 47.42 (2011) and 44.71 (2015).

"Voice and Accountability" captures perceptions of the extent to which a country's citizens are able to participate in selecting their government, as well as freedom of expression, freedom of association, and a free media. Percentile ranks indicate the country's rank among all countries covered by the aggregate indicator, with 0 corresponding to lowest rank, and 100 to highest rank. In "Voice and Accountability", Colombia scored a percentile rank of: 29.33 (1996), 34.13 (2003), 46.48 (2011) and 45.81 (2015).

See http://info.worldbank.org/governance/wgi/#reports

Despite these improvements in recent years, analysts have argued that the various threats faced by Colombia have undermined the legitimacy of state institutions. This in turn can explain much of the current configuration of Colombian politics and the poor institutional performance of key bodies, including the legislature, which has been characterised as highly fragmented and decentralized (Pachón and Johnson 2016; Botero et al. 2010; Bejarano and Pizarro 2002).

The chapter examines evidence use in a fragmented and conflict-riven political environment such as Colombia, focussing on the long-standing and highly politicised attempts to reform the Colombian health system. It shows that policy relevant evidence has consistently been used to inform and provide the rationale for draft laws submitted to Congress over the period of the reforms and appropriate and robust research had indeed entered onto policy making agenda and was cited in the legislation examined. However, reflecting the role of the legislature in the highly contested political system and the health policy subsystem, evidence was not able to change actors' initial positions and opinions and thus, political consensus on the direction of reforms could not be forged on the basis of the evidence cited. Thus while the importance of evidence to both the substance and politics of the proposed reforms was acknowledged, the inability of policy relevant evidence to overcome political divisions and form the basis of political compromise and consensus is also clear. The analysis presented here supports the conclusion that, in highly contested and fragmented political environments, evidence tends to be secondary to other political and ideological factors influencing policy change. The chapter focuses on the reform process of the Colombian health system and the uptake of research within draft laws submitted to the Colombian Parliament between 1993 and 2016.

METHODOLOGY

This chapter draws on data generated from an analysis of draft laws which are available in the public domain as well as from data gathered from semi-structured interviews with policy actors in Colombia. As in many countries, Colombia has a hierarchical legal structure with the constitution on top, followed by laws produced by the Congress, which can be Statutory laws (*leyes estatutarias*), Organic laws (*leyes orgánicas*) and Ordinary laws (*leyes ordinarias*) (Vanegas 2012). Any draft law in Colombia has to have an introductory preamble (*exposición de motivos*) which explains the nature and scope of the problem that it aims to tackle, reviews the regulatory gap that it aims to fill and presents the broad content of the law. It is in the introductory preamble of draft laws where research, if it has been reviewed to formulate the policy proposal, will be referred to. Thus, an analysis of the evidence cited in the introductory preambles allows us to examine whether research evidence has been at all up taken during the policy formulation phase and the body of research which had informed the wider policy debates.

As detailed in Annex 1, 62 draft laws were identified and selected which were then reviewed independently by the present authors of this chapter to assess whether they cited evidence to sustain their policy proposals and, if so, which type of evidence was considered. The criteria used for this assessment was whether the draft law included: (i) data produced by government and its agencies and/or academic studies to consistently define the nature and scope of the problem; and/or (ii) existing national and international research (i.e. international organizations reports, research published in peer-review journals, etc.) to sustain policy proposals. This research, however, did not seek to evaluate the "quality" of the evidence considered and eventually taken up in the draft laws.

We conducted a total of 26 interviews in Colombia in February 2014. Respondents included policy advisers and civil servants at the national level, interest groups representatives, academics, health policy experts and commentators. Through the interviews, we sought to understand the structure and of recent health policy debates in the country and the type of evidence discussed within the policy making processes. In particular, we sought to identify the factors and conditions which helped or hindered the use of evidence to inform those decisions. Interview responses were triangulated with the analysis of draft laws described above and a wider review of relevant policy reports and government documents. To ensure anonymity of respondents we refer to interviews by number. Where it is essential to the understanding or evidentiary weight of quotations, the sector from which respondents came will be detailed. Quotes in Spanish from the interviews and from other bibliographical sources were translated into English by the authors.

The Role of the Legislature in Colombia

The current institutional configuration of the Colombian state is defined by the Constitution of 1991. Colombia is a presidential system in which the President of the Republic is elected directly by the citizens for a set period of four years. The Colombian Parliament is formed of a bicameral Congress with a Senate (*Senado*), and a Chamber of Representatives (*Cámara de Representantes*), elected also for a four year period via a proportional representation system. The political party system is weak: parties do not have strong bureaucracies and structures, and are dependent instead upon individual leaders who act as figureheads, tying together otherwise loosely connected political allegiances. Under the current Constitution, the two-party system that had dominated politics prior to the 1990s was replaced by a highly fragmented, multi-party system, with later reforms, in 2003, aimed at reducing this fragmentation. The present system is characterised not only by weak party structures (with parties serving as electoral vehicles for candidates to promote their own personal agendas), but by high electoral volatility, whereby new parties frequently emerge but often cease to exist in one or two elections cycles (Botero et al. 2011; Milanese 2011; Pachón and Johnson 2016).

Within this institutional architecture, what is the role of the legislature in the policy process in Colombia? Saiegh (2010) has suggested a number of factors that can drive a legislature's policymaking role: (a) the extent of its formal powers; (b) the amount of political space/discretion afforded by other power holders, mainly the Executive branch; (c) the capacity afforded by its procedures, structures and support; and (d) the goals of members and leaders of the legislature body itself. The following section explores how these factors combine to grant a specific role to the Colombian legislature in policy making.

First, the Colombia legislature performs both traditional parliamentary roles of developing legislation and scrutinizing government through both chambers of Congress – the Senate (*Senado*), and the Chamber of Representatives (*Cámara de Representantes*) – which have largely symmetrical roles and powers. Each chamber is divided into a number of commissions which deal with specific policy matters. For example, the First Commissions of Senate and Chamber of Representatives deal with 'constitutional, ethnic and peace' matters, while the Seventh Commissions of Senate and Chamber of Representatives discuss 'health, social security, housing' issues, etc. New draft laws are registered in one of the Chambers or in both (twin projects) and are allocated to a specific Committee of that Chamber for analysis and discussion.[2]

---

[2] At registering in Congress, the project law receives a number, which different for each chamber, and thus is known by such code, the year of registration and a S or C letter depend-

Second, regarding the power of the legislature *vis-à-vis* the President of the Republic, the 1991 "constitution strengthened the checks and balances of the political system in an effort to endow political institutions with greater legitimacy after decades of limited participation and low representation" (Cárdenas et al. 2008: 202). This meant that "the president lost some capacity as an agenda-setter relative to the previous period, while congress and the constitutional court gained relative power" (Cárdenas et al. 2008: 202). However, the President of the Republic in Colombia continues to be extremely powerful within the Colombian system; enjoying several key powers to influence the legislation and the wider political process (including urgency message; legislative decrees; capacity to veto Congress projects; freedom to initiate laws in key policy areas, which are detailed below) (Saiegh 2010). The role of the President was further strengthened during the administration of President Álvaro Uribe Vélez (2002–2010), who succeeded in pushing through reforms to allow him (and future Presidents) to be re-elected for a second term. Among Latin American countries, Colombia (together with Chile, Brazil and Ecuador) grants the greatest legislative powers to presidents vis-a-vis legislatures (Saiegh 2010). However, the position of the President (and by extension, the executive) versus the legislative branch should not be overstated (Saiegh 2010). It is not "imperial presidency" but rather "limited centralism" (Milanese 2011) as the President is obliged to seek compromises with parliamentarians in order to secure the passage of legislation.

Third, law making processes in Colombia are highly institutionalised. All laws, must undergo the same basic process. The first step is that the draft law is published in the official congress bulletin (*Gaceta del Congreso*). The process starts either in the Senate or in the Chamber of Representatives, depending on which chamber the draft was first registered. This first debate occurs in the permanent commission of the chamber after which it is voted on. If it's approved it moves on to the plenary of the chambers. Once the plenary has approved the draft is sent to the remaining chamber's permanent commission to be debated, voted and if successful, passed to the plenary. If there are differences between the approved texts in each chamber, a conciliatory draft is produced by an appointed group consisting

ing on whether it refers to the Senate or the Chamber of Representatives. For example, the Statutory Law Project (Proyecto Ley Estatutaria, PLE) registration in Senate was PLE209/2013S and its Congress twin-project is PLE267/2013C – this is represented in this chapter in the following way: PLE209/2013S [+ PLE267/2013C].

of an equal number of members of each chamber. Finally, the draft requires the President's signature to enter into law. In the case of statutory laws (and those issued under any of the extraordinary procedures), review by the Constitutional Court is required before the President's signature.

The regulations governing Congress allow for a series of extraordinary procedures to deal with specific situations. One of them is an "urgency message" whereby the President requests a higher priority be assigned to a draft law in an expedited process which should last no more than 30 days in each Chamber. The procedure means deliberation and voting on the proposed law are conducted jointly between the Commissions of the Senate and the Chamber of Representatives. Then, the draft statutory law is voted separately by each Chamber on a plenary session. A final "conciliatory" draft is produced and reviewed by the Constitutional Court to confirm that the legislation enacted is compatible with the Constitution, before being signed into by the President of the Republic. The high turnover of MPs and the weak party structures limit the institutional knowledge and technical capacity of the legislative branch in Colombia (Scartascini 2008: 47). There is very low party discipline and party leaders have only limited control of the legislative agenda (Pachón and Johnson 2016).

Finally, one of the most prominent elements of Colombia's legislature is the "personalist" nature of political candidacies (Pachón and Hoskin 2011), in which political parties serve mainly as conduits for prominent individuals, in a system favouring 'client' relations over partisan identities (Saiegh 2010; Milanese 2011; Pachón and Johnson 2016; also confirmed in interviews). Often, this involves prioritizing what Pachón and Johnson (2016) have called "distributive pork-barrel projects": obtaining resources to benefit the constituency that gets them elected (see also Milanese 2011). Saiegh (2010) highlights in addition that "legislators orientate towards satisfying narrow geographic interests". National policy makers are discouraged from making radical reforms through Congress which may affected established networks of vested interest and reforms are instead passed incrementally through executive decrees [Interview 8] or brought about through rulings of the Constitutional Court on the provision of health services (see Hawkins and Alvarez Rosete 2017).

The core of the legislature's activity is also not directed by party groups but by the Commissions of the Chamber of Representatives and the Senate, which are not under the control of party leaders but exercise significant control over the Congressional agenda (Pachón and Johnson 2016). Since the Commissions in Colombia constitute the first stage of bill approval, they "can prevent bills from ever getting to the floor. This contrasts with the situation of most legislatures in Latin America, in which committees only advise the floor with positive or negative reports" (Pachón and Johnson 2016: 73). Thus, legislators seek election to key Commissions, i.e. those which allocate resources or which play key gatekeeping functions, such as Commissions I of the Congress and the Senate in ballots held amongst parliamentarians on the first day of the legislature term (Pachón and Johnson 2016). This may mean competing for seats with members of the same party while getting support from other political groups, and again reflects the personalist, highly fragmented and decentralised nature of the Colombian legislature. Consequently, the Colombian legislature is not an arena which facilitates consensus building and constructive approaches to policymaking, with clear implications for evidence use.

COLOMBIA'S HIGHLY CONTESTED HEALTH POLICY SUBSYSTEM

The divisions and fragmentation in Colombian society and politics are reflected in its health policy debates. The health system has suffered from a lack of fundamental consensus over its most basic organising principles and structures since its inception with the passage of Law 100 in 1993. This lack of consensus has continued throughout the almost constant process of reform which the system has undergone. Despite successive proposals for reform, high levels of political contestation have resulted in policy stasis. Deep ideological disagreements have been sustained on issues such as the financing of the system (insurance versus taxation based models); the involvement of private sector providers; and whether limits should be placed to the right to health care. This reform process reflects in part the role played by competing coalitions of actors present within the Colombian health sector, and their various attempts to shape the health system in ways amenable to their underlying interests and values. We have analysed elsewhere the interactions between three principal coalitions of actors involved in the health system reform process in the context of Colombia's antagonistic politics (Hawkins and Alvarez Rosete 2017; Álvarez and Hawkins 2018).

It is possible to identify two key phases in the health system reform process. In the first phase (1993–2010), a "dominant" coalition of government technocrats, congressmen, insurance companies, the financial sector and the private health providers (including the pharmaceutical companies) emerged and was able to shape the health policy agenda. Between 2003 and 2009, under the administration of President Uribe, a set of actors began to emerge which sought to challenge the dominant coalition but were not at this juncture effectively coordinated as a coalition of actors, and so no solid agreements on a shared policy agenda between different groups were reached.

The second phase began under the current Presidency of Juan Manuel Santos in 2010 and is still ongoing. This chapter analyses the period up to 2016. A gradual coalescing of actors into distinct advocacy coalitions, increasingly coordinated and mobilised around shared beliefs and policy solutions, began to challenge those of the "dominant coalition". The emergence of "challenging" coalitions occurred in parallel with the weakening of the "dominant coalition" and the gradually weakening relationships between this coalition and successive Ministers of Health. However, as the recent passage of Statutory Law 1751 – which confirmed the principles and values of the existing health system, whilst clarifying the rights and responsibilities of patients – demonstrated, the two challenger coalitions of actors have not been powerful enough to override the hegemony of the dominant coalition and cross-coalition agreements have not been achieved.

EVIDENCE USE IN THE FIRST PHASE OF HEALTH REFORM (1992–2010)

Law 100 of 1993, which set up the current health system, was passed during the government of President César Gaviria (1990–1994), in the context of a wider programme of the state reforms, which included the enactment of a new constitution in July 1991 (Vega-Vargas et al. 2012; González-Rosetti and Bossert 2000; Jaramillo 1998). As mentioned above, these political reforms had strengthened the power of Congress, so that it was able to impose policy initiatives on the Executive, including health reforms (González-Rosetti and Bossert 2000: 24). As González-Rosetti and Bossert comment (2000: 26): "The health reform was not part of [President Gaviria's] initial policy agenda, which focused on the social security reform. Instead, it was the concession the Executive had to make to Congress in order to have the pension reform approved." Indeed, the first version of Project Law PL155/1992S submitted to Senate by the Executive in September 1992 (and its twin draft law in the Chamber of Representatives PL204/1992C), which eventually became Law 100 later in 1993, proposed reforms of the pension system but did not include health, so Commission VII of the Senate vetoed the draft and requested the government to adopt a comprehensive approach to social security reform which also included the health system (Uribe 2009). At that time, the Minister of Health was Gustavo de Roux, who belonged to the centre-left party the *Alianza Democrática M-19* and whose ideas on the health reforms were not aligned with President Gaviria's view.

In November 1992, de Roux was replaced by Juan Luis Londoño, who had been deputy director of the National Planning Department (*Departamento Nacional de Planeación*) and who assembled a small group of national experts to take the reform task forward, supported by the group of international consultants of the Colombia Health Sector Reform Project of the Harvard School of Public Health (Bossert et al. 1998). In that same month, Londoño submitted to Congress an addition to PL155/1992S which proposed the setting up of a subsidised health scheme for the poor; but it was again vetoed by the Commission VII of the Senate, which argued again that this was only a partial reform to the health sector (Uribe 2009).

Thus, the process of negotiations on different policy options started again and a number of parties and pressure groups presented legislative projects during the first months of 1993 (Uribe 2009). These proposals were considered by a group of experts, which, under the coordination of Londoño's team, produced a new version of PL155/1992S, which was registered in Congress in April 1993. As Glassman et al. (2009: 7) state, with this proposal "[t]he administration committed to accelerating the expansion of subsidized health insurance for the poor; developing a program to support the redesign, reorganization and modernization of public hospitals and to ensure their financial sustainability; and strengthening the national immunization program." This version of PL155/1992S passed quickly through Congress between May and December, becoming Law 100 on 23 December 1993.

Key characteristics of the Colombian legislature discussed above are evident in the process of legislating the PL155/1992S into Law 100 of 1993. First, discussions within the legislature took place and a wide range of stakeholders had the opportunity to present proposals and put forward policy demands. Whilst the policy initiative came from the executive, the legislature became the central arena for these policy discussions. Indeed, the legislature managed to influence significantly the final outcome of the policy process (Uribe 2009). The vetoes to two government's versions of PL 155/1992S within Commission VII confirms Saiegh's (2010) assertion that legislatures can be active players in policy making by being blunt veto players, forcing the executive to take alternative paths.

Second, this process also shows that the different policy proposals were not submitted by the political parties with representation in the legislature, but by individual congressmen representing interest groups or social movements. This reflects Colombia's weak party system and the "personalist" nature of political candidacies explained above.

Third, evidence from scientific research was available to (and thus potentially used by) decision makers and legislators. On the executive side in particular, the consultancy team from the Harvard School of Public Health provided a continuous flow of information and knowledge at demand from Londoño and his team. According to one of our interviewees, Londoño did not want "one-off consultancy" but continuous support in designing and implementing the law and in providing answers to policy questions [Interview 8]. Research produced by academic institutions and think tanks (i.e. Fedesarrollo) was also available to other key participants of the policy process.

As an attempt to generate knowledge to support the implementation of Law 100, the government set up the Program for Supporting the Health Reform (*Programa de Apoyo a la Reforma de Salud*, PARS) in 1996 with the financial and technical support of the Inter-American Development Bank. The Program aimed to provide technical assistance and capacity building, to produce specialised research and strategies to transfer such knowledge to decision-makers at the Ministry of Health. More than 100 analytical studies and consultancy projects were developed until the programme finished in 2008 (MPS and Gesaworld 2008). Alongside the PARS, the strategic policy documents produced by the National Council of Economic and Social Policies (*Consejo Nacional de Políticas Económicas y Sociales*, CONPES)[3] on specific economic and social policy areas became a key tool to support decision making at the national level.

Despite these efforts, by 2001 the health system was facing a "severe and generalized financial crisis" leading to successive attempts to address these through reforms (Glassman et al. 2009: 7). A first wave of legislation designed to reform the health system was submitted to Congress in 2003 and 2004, but none of it was ultimately passed (Hernández 2005). The first was draft law proposed to reform Law 100 was PL180/2004S, to which other projects such as PL236/2004S and PL241/2004S were latter added for joint discussion in Congress. Supporting evidence does not appear prominently in the preambles of the draft laws, with the exception

---

[3] DNP website, https://www.dnp.gov.co/CONPES/DocumentosConpes.aspx

of PL180/2004s. However, the evidence is cited only in passing and without an attempt to detailed engagement. The legislative term closed in June 2004 without these draft laws having progressed, and so they were abandoned (Hernández 2005).

In 2004, a second wave of 14 draft laws was submitted to Congress, starting with PL19/2004S and followed by others such as PL31/2004S and PL33/2004S. These and the rest of the 14-strong list were accumulated to the PL52/2004S submitted by the government for parliamentary discussion. These stalled in Congress, where health insurers managed to orchestrate strong opposition, with the support of the Ministry of Finance. Furthermore, other legislative priorities such as pension reform and legislation to allow the re-election of President Uribe relegated the importance of PL52/2004S, and it was ultimately abandoned (Guzmán 2006). Three of these draft laws– (PL52/2004S, PL31/2004S and PL33/2004S) did include discussion of relevant supporting evidence. Although watered down in terms of scope and depth of the reforms it proposed, PL52/2004S was well supported by research evidence, including most recent data from the 2003 National Health Survey (*Encuesta Nacional de Salud*), the Quality of Life National Survey (*Encuesta Nacional de Calidad de Vida*) and the 2004 CONPES document on social policy issues. More prominently, PL31/2004S made use of extensive evidence from various sources: it brought in data from a 2003 CONPES and other official statistics (i.e. Ministry of Social Protection, SIVIGILA) as well as data from Pan-American Health Organization (PAHO) studies, the PARS studies, etc. National and international statistics were also referred to in PL33/2004S.

No further legislative initiatives were reintroduced in Congress until the summer 2006. The beginning of a new legislative term saw the registration of PL40/2006S in Senate [the twin draft law in Chamber of Representatives was PL2/2006C] to which 16 other draft laws – many registered by individual legislators – were progressively accumulated. Of all these draft laws, only two – PL116/2006S and PL122/2006S – drew on official statistics and linked arguments to published research, to sustain their proposals while the twin draft laws [PL40/2006S + PL2/2006C] registered by Minister of Social Protection, Diego Palacio, were not firmly grounded relevant evidence. PL40/2006S [+PL2/2006C] and its accumulated projects were discussed over the second half of 2006 and approved in a joint commission debate in December, leading to the passage of Law 1122 on 9 January 2007. The scope and aim of Law 1122 ultimately became to strengthen system regulations and de-judicialise health care, i.e. the *tutela* system of protection writs through which citizens are able to seek access to health service via the courts (for a more detailed discussion of *tutelas* and the effects of judicialisation on evidence use see Hawkins and Alvarez Rosete 2017) (Restrepo 2007; Bernal et al. 2012: 25). Law 1122 led to the creation of the Regulatory Commission for Health (*Comisión de Regulación en Salud, CRES*), a decision-making body at arm's length affiliated to the Ministry of Health, with the role of updating the basket of benefits through the use of high quality evidence and a strong and transparent decision-making methodology. The creation of the CRES reveals the attempt to bring more evidence into the policy making process, although this too would be subject to later reform.

Ultimately, all these initiatives to address the sustainability of the health system stalled and "by the end of the decade, the health system was in deep crisis" (Bernal et al. 2012: 25) and with seemingly little prospect of reform. Scientific research was available to policy makers in Colombia and even informed the different draft laws submitted to Congress between 1993 and 2010. However, none of these draft laws was able to pass successfully through Congress. This suggests that while evidence was important in informing policy debates, and proposed legislation, it was unable, in the context of deep politicization and embedded vested interests, to bring about effective reforms of health system and to relieve the mounting pressures it faced.

EVIDENCE USE IN SECOND PHASE OF HEALTH REFORMS (2010–2016)

In the last month of President Uribe's Presidency in July 2010, draft law PL01/2010S was registered in the Senate [along with its twin draft in the Chamber of Representatives PL106/2010C]. President Santos replaced Uribe as President with proposals for an ambitious programme of state reforms, to align the public administration with the goals of the 2010–2014 National Development Plan (Strazza 2014). The reforms transformed the centre of government in Colombia and resulted in a step change in the availability of policy-relevant evidence, and the concern with evidence use in health policy making.

Draft laws PL1/2010S [+PL106/2010C] were discussed alongside another 10 draft laws accumulated to it, leading to the passage of Law 1438 in January 2011. Only the preamble of PL01/2010S included references to evidence. Nevertheless, Law 1438 regulated the setting up of the Institute of Health Technology Assessment (*Instituto de Evaluación de Tecnologías Sanitarias*, IETS), which was established in September 2012 and, only a few months later, in December 2012, the CRES was abolished and the Ministry of Health "re-assumed its role of resource-allocation decision-maker" (Castro 2014: 22, 131). As Dargent (2015) notes, the Santos reforms led experts and technocrats to "regain salience" at the Ministry of Health. According to Minister of Health Gaviria, the Ministry is now "a technocratic fortress", in which "decisions are now made independently of electoral politics" (Gaviria 2015). Whilst decision making of this kind is never completely apolitical, these claims speak to but a desire to introduce evidence into the decision making process more systematically and the potential for this to rationalise decision making processes.

During the second half of 2010 a new wave of reforms were introduced to Congress by different parliamentarians. Four draft statutory laws – PLE186/2010S and the accumulated draft laws PLE189/2010S, PLE131/2010C and PLE198/2010S – which aimed to define "the essential core of the right to health" were discussed in Parliament. Research evidence was provided in the preambles of 3 of the 4 draft laws submitted to Congress. PLE186/2010S analyses in detail the dramatic increase of health care costs and its causes, while PLE189/2010S included an extensive commentary on the vision and recommendations of the World Health Report 2008 on primary care (WHR 2008). PLE198/2010S provided figures on equity and access to health services based upon official statistics, for example, and includes references to specialised literature to back up the proposals suggested. All these draft laws however did not complete the process in a single legislature and hence had to be abandoned.

A new window of opportunity for policy change opened up in the summer of 2012 with the submission to Congress of four draft statutory laws (PLE48/2012S; PLE59/2012C; PLE105/2012S; and PLE112/2012S) and one ordinary draft law (PL51/2012S, which was consequently accumulated to PL210/2013S which came later). Of the four statutory laws, PLE48/2012S was informed by good quality research obtained from international comparisons, published studies and interviews with experts. PLE105/2012S and PLE112/2012S also referenced publications and official data, while PLE59/2012C did not mention any specific research.

With the impetus brought by the newly appointed Health Minister Gaviria, the government sought to take the initiative on the reform of the health system and develop both a Statutory Law and an Ordinary Law. On 19 March 2013, the government registered two draft reform laws in Parliament: President Santos registered the draft Statutory Law PLE 209/2013S at the Senate [and twin project PLE267/2013C at the Chamber] and Minister Gaviria registered the draft Ordinary Law PL210/2013S at the

Senate [and its twin project PL147/2013C at the Chamber]. Both PLE209/2013S [+PLE267/2013C] discussed in Commission I and PL210/2013S [+PL147/2013C] discussed in Commission VII were supported by extensive official statistics and underpinned arguments on published research.

Draft Statutory Law PLE209/2013S was enacted on 16 February 2015, became Statutory Law 1751. However, Ordinary Draft law PL210/2013S could not to be approved within two legislative periods and hence was abandoned. The re-election of President Santos in May 2014, and the continuation in office of Minister of Health Gaviria, presented a second opportunity to pass legislation in a new legislative period. A new draft law PL77/2014S was registered on 29 August 2014 to bring back some of the financial instruments considered in the failed PL210/2013S. Thus, PL77/2014S got accumulated to PL24/2014S [+PL109/2015C]. However, none of the proposed laws referred to scientific evidence in their preambles. After a long legislative process, the project was finally passed as Law 1797 on 13 July 2016.

Conclusion

The analysis of the more than 20-year long process of reforming Law 100 shows that evidence can, and indeed did, inform health policies in a highly contested and fragmented political setting. The analysis of draft laws designed to reform the health system shows that policy relevant evidence was available to actors involved in reforming the health system and was used to inform a number of key draft laws submitted to parliament. We identified high levels of contestation and fragmentation at different levels of Colombian society: the social, political and policy levels, which provide the institutional context in which policy problems emerge and policy actors seek to address them. In this context, the availability of policy relevant evidence offers a potential means of circumventing and overcoming, political fragmentation and contestation. However, the deep seated nature of the vested interests in the Colombian health system and the health systems models which they favoured, meant that reform proposals were often stymied. Whilst it is not possible to depoliticize or solve policy dilemmas through recourse to evidence alone, it is possible, at times, to use evidence as a means of generating consensus or providing the impetus towards compromise. To overcome the endemic problems of weak political and legislative structures, and engrained political cleavages, new bodies were formed which were tasked with the collection, interpretation and deployment of policy relevant evidence.

However, despite the institutionalised mechanisms of evidence generation and synthesis, the translation of research into policy and legislation remained limited and piecemeal. Many draft laws provided only minimal data on the extent of the problems facing the health system in Colombia, and their reform proposals were mostly based upon general commentaries of the functioning and challenges of the system (i.e. PL229/2010S; PLE59/2012C; PL51/2012S; PL233/2013S; etc.). A small number of other draft laws, which quoted academic studies to back up their analysis of the extent of the problem, tended however to refer to a biased selection of studies (that is, research which would fit their ideological stances; i.e. PLE105/2012S; PLE112/2012S). However, those draft laws submitted by the government, especially during the last phase of the reform, included extended empirical and analytical sections. For example, the PLE209/2013S and PL210/2013S provide a deep and wide analysis of the problems of the Colombian health system.

Reflecting the role of the legislature in Colombia's highly contested political system and health policy subsystem, evidence cited in draft laws was unable to forge consensus amongst relevant policy actors over the direction of the health system reforms. The deep confrontations within the Colombian legislature did not facilitate political agreements nor play a constructive role in health policymaking. Scientific research was available and at the disposal of legislators, but it was unable to provide the common ground on which to overcome embedded policy positions and form the basis of compromise over the direction of health systems reforms.

Annex 1: Laws and Draft Laws Reviewed

underlined = *preamble refers to/quotes research*

1992–2010

1993–2002

- *PLs that led to Law 100:* PL155/1992S [+PL204/1992C]

2003–2004

- PL180/2004S and accumulated: PL236/2004S; PL238/2004S; PL241/2004S; PL242/2004S

- PL52/2004S and accumulated: PL19/2004S; PL31/2004S; PL33/2004S; PL38/2004S; PL54/2004; PL57/2004S; PL58/2004S; PL98/2004S; PL105/2004S; PL115/2004S; PL122/2004S; PL151/2004S

2006–2007

- *PLs that led to Law 1122:* PL40/2006S [+PL2/2006C] and accumulated PL20/2006S; PL26/2006S; PL38/2006S; PL67/2006S; PL116/2006S; PL122/2006S; PL128/2006S; PL143/2006S; PL1/2006C; PL18/2006C; PL84/2006C; PL130/2006C; PL137/2006C; PL140/2006C; PL141/2006C and PL1/2006S [+PL87/2006C]

2010–2016

2010

- *PLs that led to Law 1438:* PL1/2010S [+PL106/2010C] and accumulated: PL95/2010S; PL143/2010S; PL147/2010S; PL160/2010S; PL161/2010S; PL182/2010S; PL87/2010C, PL35/2010C; PL111/2010C; PL126/2010C
- PLE186/2010S and accumulated: PLE189/2010S; PLE131/2010C; PLE198/2010S
- PL229/2010S

2012

- PLE48/2012S and accumulated: PLE59/2012C; PLE105/2012S; PLE112/2012S;

2013–2014

- *PLEs that led to Law 1751:* PLE209/2013S [+PLE267/2013C]
- PL210/2013S [+PL147/2013C] and accumulated: PL233/2013S; PL51/2012S

2014–2016

- *PLs that led to Law 1797:* PL77/2014S and accumulated PL24/2014S [+PL109/2015C]

References

Álvarez-Rosete, A, and B. Hawkins. 2018. Advocacy coalitions, contestation and policy stasis: The twenty year reform process of the Colombian health system. *Latin American Policy.* Available at: https://doi.org/10.1111/psj.12230.

Bejarano, A.M., and E. Pizarro Leóngómez. 2002. From *"restricted" to "besieged": The changing nature of the limits to democracy in Colombia*, Working Paper #296, The Helen Kellogg Institute for International Studies. Available at https://kellogg.nd.edu/publications/workingpapers/WPS/296.pdf

Bernal, O., J.C. Forero, and I. Forde. 2012. Colombia's response to crisis. *British Medical Journal* 344: 25–27.

Bossert, T., W. Hsiao, M. Barrera, L. Alarcon, M. Leo, and C. Casares. 1998. Transformation of ministries of health in the era of health reform: The case of Colombia. *Health Policy and Planning* 13 (1): 59–77.

Botero, F., G.W. Hoskin, and M. Pachón. 2010. Sobre forma y sustancia: una evaluación de la democracia electoral en Colombia. *Revista de Ciencia Política* 30 (1): 41–64.

Botero F., R. Losada, and L. Wills. 2011. Sistema de partidos en Colombia 1974–2010: ¿la evolución hacia el multipartidismo?, *Seminario sobre Estabilidad y Cambio del Sistema de Partidos en América Latina [GIPSAL]*, December 1. Available at: http://americo.usal.es/iberoame/sites/default/files/botero_losada_wills_colombia.pdf

Cárdenas M., R. Junguito, and M. Pachón. 2008. Political institutions and policy outcomes in Colombia: The effects of the 1991 constitution. In *Policymaking in Latin America: how politics shapes policies*, ed. E. Stein and M. Tommasi with P. Spiller and C. Scartascini, 199–242. Washington, DC/Cambridge, MA: Inter-American Development Bank & David Rockefeller Center for Latin American Studies.

Castro, H. 2014. *Assessing the feasibility of conducting and using health technology assessment in Colombia. The case of severe haemophilia A.* Unpublished doctoral thesis, London: London School of Hygiene and Tropical Medicine, University of London.

Dargent, E. 2015. *Technocracy and democracy in Latin America: The experts running government.* Cambridge: Cambridge University press.

Gaviria A. 2015. Hoy puedo decir con orgullo que Minsalud es un fortín tecnocrático, *El Tiempo*, January 4. Available at http://www.eltiempo.com/estilo-de-vida/salud/hoy-puedo-decir-con-orgullo-que-minsalud-es-un-fortin-tecnocratico/15050215

Glassman, A.L., J.L. Escobar, A. Giuffrida, and U. Giedion, eds. 2009. *From few to many. Ten years of health insurance expansion in Colombia.* Washington, DC: Inter-American Development Bank and The Brookings Institution.

González-Rosetti, A., and T.J. Bossert. 2000. *Enhancing the political feasibility of health reform: A comparative analysis of Chile, Colombia, and Mexico.* LAC Health Sector Reform Initiative 36. Boston: United States Agency for International Development and Harvard School of Public Health.

Guzmán, H. 2006. Fracasó el proyecto de ley 52: la gran estafa. El Pulso. *Periódico para el sector de la salud* 7 (94). Available at http://www.periodicoelpulso.com/html/jul06/general/general-13.htm

Hawkins, B., and A. Alvarez Rosete 2017. Judicialization and health policy in Colombia: The implications for evidence-informed policymaking. *Policy Studies Journal.* Available at: http://onlinelibrary.wiley.com/doi/10.1111/psj.12230/full

Hernández Álvarez, M. 2005. Propuestas de reforma a la ley 100 de 1993. Opciones sociopolíticas en debate, Revista Gerencia y Políticas de Salud, no. 9, December, 180–190.

Jaramillo-Pérez, I. 1998. *El Futuro de la Salud en Colombia.* Bogotá: Tercer Mundo Editores.

Kim, J.Y. 2016. Op-Ed by World Bank Group President Jim Yong Kim: Colombia's peace can lead to inclusive economic growth, September 26. The World Bank. Available at http://www.worldbank.org/en/news/opinion/2016/09/26/op-ed-colombias-peace-can-lead-to-inclusive-economic-growth

Milanese, J.P. 2011. Participación, éxito y prioridad. Un análisis macro de los equilibrios en las relaciones entre los poderes ejecutivo y legislativo en Colombia, 2002–2006. CS, 8, 111–145.

Ministerio de Protección Social (MPS) and Gesaworld. 2008. De la generación de conocimiento a la formulación de políticas públicas. *Evaluación externa del PARS 1996–2007,* Bogotá: Programa de Apoyo a la Reforma de Salud. Available at: https://www.minsalud.gov.co/Documentos%20y%20Publicaciones/EVALUACION%20EXTERNA.pdf

Pachón, M., and G. Hoskin. 2011. Colombia 2010: An analysis of the legislative and presidential elections. *Colombia International* 74: 9–26.

Pachón, M., and G.B. Johnson. 2016. When's the party (or coalition)? Agenda setting in a highly fragmented, decentralized legislatura. *Journal of Politics in Latin America* 2: 71–100.

Restrepo, J.H. 2007. ¿Qué cambió en la seguridad social con la Ley 1122? *Revista de Facultad Nacional de Salud Pública* 25 (1): 82–89.

Saiegh, S.M. 2010. Active players or rubber stamps? An evaluation of the policy-making role of Latin American legislatures. In *How democracy works. Political institutions, actors and arenas in Latin American Policymaking,* ed. C. Scartascini, E. Stein, and M. Tommasi, 47–75. Washington, DC/Cambridge, MA: Inter-American Development Bank & David Rockefeller Center for Latin American Studies.

Scartascini, C. 2008. Who's who in the PMP: An overview of actors, incentives, and the roles they play. In *Policymaking in Latin America: How politics shapes policies,* ed. E. Stein and M. Tommasi with P. Spiller and C. Scartascini, 29–68. Washington, DC/Cambridge, MA: Inter-American Development Bank and David Rockefeller Center for Latin American Studies.

Strazza, L. 2014. *Diagnóstico institucional del servicio civil en América Latina: Colombia*, Banco Interamericano de Desarrollo.
Uribe Gómez MM. 2009. *La contienda por las reformas del sistema de salud en Colombia (1990–2006)*. Doctoral thesis. México: Universidad Nacional Autónoma de México. Available at: http://ces.colmex.mx/pdfs/tesis/tesis_uribe_gomez.pdf
Vanegas Gil, P. 2012. Las leyes estatutarias en el ordenamiento jurídico colombiano: un ejemplo de rigidez normativa. *Revista Médico Legal* 13, 2.
Vega-Vargas, M., J.C. Eslava-Castañeda, D. Arrubla-Sánchez, and M. Hernández-Álvarez. 2012. La reforma sanitaria en la Colombia de finales del siglo XX: aproximación histórica desde el análisis sociopolítico. *Revista Gerencia y Políticas de Salud* 11 (23): 58–84.
World Health Report (WHR). 2008. Primary health care (now more than ever). Geneva: World health Organization. Available at http://www.who.int/whr/2008/en/

Open Access This chapter is licensed under the terms of the Creative Commons Attribution 4.0 International License (http://creativecommons.org/licenses/by/4.0/), which permits use, sharing, adaptation, distribution and reproduction in any medium or format, as long as you give appropriate credit to the original author(s) and the source, provide a link to the Creative Commons license and indicate if changes were made.

The images or other third party material in this chapter are included in the chapter's Creative Commons license, unless indicated otherwise in a credit line to the material. If material is not included in the chapter's Creative Commons license and your intended use is not permitted by statutory regulation or exceeds the permitted use, you will need to obtain permission directly from the copyright holder.

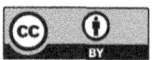

CHAPTER 6

The Politics of Evidence Use in Health Policy Making in Germany: The Case of Regulating Hospital Minimum Volumes

Stefanie Ettelt

INTRODUCTION

In Germany, the idea of evidence-based policy as a model of modern policy-making has not engendered as much enthusiasm as in other countries, particularly in the Anglo-Saxon world (Jun and Grabow 2008; Knieps 2009). German policy-makers and researchers are broadly in agreement that scientific evidence has become more relevant to policy-making over time to address increasingly complex policy problems and to provide legitimacy for potentially unpopular decisions (Renn 1995; Mayntz 2009).

This chapter presents an updated version of a paper first published as:
Ettelt, S. 2017. The politics of evidence use in health policy making in Germany – The case of regulating hospital minimum volumes. *Journal of Health Politics, Policy and Law* 42 (3): 513–538.

S. Ettelt (✉)
London School of Hygiene and Tropical Medicine, London, UK
e-mail: stefanie.ettelt@lshtm.ac.uk

© The Author(s) 2018
J. Parkhurst et al. (eds.), *Evidence Use in Health Policy Making*,
International Series on Public Policy,
https://doi.org/10.1007/978-3-319-93467-9_6

There is also an ever growing demand for expertise met by an array of scientific advisory committees, research institutes, expert commissions and expert networks providing advice to government (Kloten 2006; Siefken 2007; Jun and Grabow 2008; Blum and Schubert 2013). This is particularly visible in health care policy, in which scientific evidence use has become institutionally embedded, for example, through the creation of the Institute for Quality and Efficiency in Health Care (*Institut für Qualität und Wirtschaftlichkeit im Gesundheitswesen*, IQWiG) (IQWiG 2015) as a provider of independent health technology assessments in the corporatist sector.

However, much scepticism about the role of scientific evidence exists outside the narrow confines of health technology assessment, with some commentators seeing references to evidence representing little more than 'scientifically cloaked lobbyism' (Knieps 2009). The complexity of the policy process in Germany – with its multitude of actors that exist within a federal, corporatist system, and the dominance of legislation over other forms of policy-making – would not lend itself to support notions of evidence-based policy.

Policy scholars have frequently noted the role of corporatism in health policy in Germany, which has given organised interests a central role in decision-making (Lehmbruch 1988; Lijphart and Crepaz 1991). The state has delegated a wide range of governance tasks to the respective associations of office-based doctors (i.e. family doctors as well as specialists), hospitals and sickness funds, which include, for example, decisions about public reimbursement of pharmaceuticals and medical services, and the definition of rules relating to quality assurance and reimbursement (Bandelow 2004). The same organised interests also have substantial influence on law making both at federal and state levels. For a long time, political parties had clear allegiances to specific interests, for example, the Social Democrats (SPD) tending to support the role of sickness funds while the Free Democrats (FDP) sought opportunities to extend the scope of private insurance, although these allegiances are not as clear as they used to be.

Provider organisations, especially those representing office-based doctors, used to be particularly influential and able to influence, and stymie, policy proposals as veto players within decision-making processes (Tsebelis 2011). Yet over the years the power dynamics between actors have changed, bringing about new patterns of organisational behaviour (Bandelow 2009). Consecutive reforms have strengthened sickness funds vis-à-vis provider organisations (e.g. by changing voting rules in committees) thus shifting the balance between payers and providers (Bandelow 2009). The federal government has also become more assertive in setting the national framework for corporatist decision-making. This was accompanied by the creation of new organisations through the merger of several associations of sickness funds into one, the *Gemeinsame Spitzenverband*, and by bringing together several committees to form the Federal Joint Committee (*Gemeinsamer Bundesausschuss*, GBA). The latter was aimed at professionalising and formalising the process of health policy-making and now forms the top decision-making body within the corporatist sector (Gerlinger 2010).

Traditional alliances have also weakened and lines of opposition have become blurred. Physicians associations now face the difficulty of representing doctors in primary and secondary care who are often pitched against each other in questions of resource allocation. Likewise, the German Hospital Association (*Deutsche Krankenhausgesellschaft*) represents all hospitals providing publicly funded services, irrespective of their size, ownership status and type of services provided. Policy changes such as the introduction of activity-based payments has also increased the competition between hospitals for patients and funding. Thus changes in policy – be they targeted at cost control or at securing quality of care – increasingly affect provider organisations in different ways, making it more difficult for top associations to present a unified front. Commentators noted that while corporatist actors still wield substantial influence, the nature of corporatism has changed over time and become more pluralist, yet also more adversarial and less consensual in style (Bandelow 2004). These dynamics also play out in the 'legalistic culture' of German policy-making, in which law-making and legal adjudication are crucial constituents of the policy process (Strueck 2013). In this chapter, it is argued that the changing style of decision-making is also demonstrated in the increased role of evidence use for both substantiating and legitimising decisions.

This chapter will explore how health policy actors in Germany have used scientific evidence to promote their aims and objectives, using the case of minimum volumes as a pertinent example. Based on the idea that quality improves with greater experience in a given procedure ('practice makes perfect'), minimum volumes have been introduced for a number of highly specialised hospital services as a measure of improving quality of care. The policy has also been introduced at the time of the formation of the GBA as the top decision making body of the self-administration in health care. Given that the latest lawsuit only concluded in December 2015 the discussion about minimum policy allows for an analysis of the role of the GBA in professionalising health policy-making, which also changed the role of scientific evidence.

The chapter will examine the role of evidence at three different stages of the policy process:

– The making of the legislative framework taking place in the two chambers of parliament, the Federal Assembly (*Bundestag*) and Federal Council (*Bundesrat*);
– The definition of minimum volumes by the 'corporatist' self-administration, represented by the GBA; and
– Legal adjudication in the social courts, charged with reviewing the legitimacy of minimum volumes set by the GBA.

It is not without irony that the idea of regulating minimum volumes as a measure of quality improvement was initially inspired by research: Studies in the United States suggested that hospitals that performed a larger number of highly complex surgeries produced better outcomes for patients than hospitals that provided these services less often (e.g. Birkmeyer et al. 1999). The idea of turning volume-outcome relationships into a policy proposal has been credited to health economist and university professor Karl Lauterbach who, at the time, was an influential policy advisory to the Federal Minister of Health Ulla Schmidt. Minimum volumes were passed into law in 2002 and have been specified and operationalised in the years that followed, attracting much controversy as well as legal challenge from hospitals.

The following section provides an introduction into the literature on strategic evidence use, followed by a description of the study methods and a summary of the scientific evidence base for minimum volumes. The middle section of the chapter is devoted to the analysis of the role of scientific evidence at different stages of the policy process. The chapter finishes with a discussion and conclusion.

Table of key organisations and committees

German	English	Function
Ausschuss Krankenhaus	Hospital Committee	Committee representing hospitals and sickness funds, mandated with decision-making for the hospital sector before 2004
Bundesrat	Federal Council	Chamber of parliament representing the governments of the states (Länder)
Bundestag	Federal Assembly	Chamber of parliament representing elected political parties
Deutsche Krankenhausgesellschaft	German Hospital Association	Federal-level association of hospitals
Gemeinsamer Bundesausschuss (GBA)	Federal Joint Committee	Top decision-making body of the corporatist self-administration in health care, since 2004
Gesundheitsausschuss	Health Committee	Parliamentary committee, preparing health related legislation for the *Bundestag*
Vermittlungsausschuss	Mediation Committee	Parliamentary committing, mediating between *Bundestag* and *Bundesrat*

STRATEGIC USES OF EVIDENCE IN HEALTH POLICY-MAKING

Carol Weiss observed in her 1979 paper that scientific evidence can be used for at least seven purposes (Weiss 1979). 'Instrumental' use is what proponents of evidence-based policy usually have in mind when they demand for research findings to be taken account of in policy decisions. However, Weiss argued that research typically influences policy in more indirect ways, with knowledge from research filtering through to policy-makers over time and in often far more convoluted ways than ideas of straight forward application would suggest. 'Political' use implies that policy-makers utilise scientific evidence in a more active manner, yet for specific, politically driven purposes. Such use, also often called 'symbolic' or 'tactical', is therefore always selective, with policy-makers choosing those pieces of evidence that best promote their case. For the purists of evidence-based policy, strategic use comes close to 'policy-based evidence', defeating the purpose of 'objective' science of making policy better informed and more rational (Marmot 2004).

However, for scholars of the policy process, selective use is by no means a surprise. Majone (1989) was one of the first to argue that evidence is typically used as a means of persuasion as part of a political argument. Greenhalgh and Russell (2007) found that evidence is often selected to fit an "argumentation game" played by policy actors by employing rhetoric and mobilising considerations of plausibility and reasonableness to achieve their aims. From that perspective, evidence use is better described as constitutive of the "social drama" of policy-making rather than seen as an end in itself. Yet there is always the question of who uses evidence strategically and for which purpose. Hind, for example, has warned that both the state and corporations use science to legitimise their actions, which in his view constitutes a serious threat to reasoning and rationality, the core values of modern societies (Hind 2007).

The role of scientific evidence in legitimising decisions has also been extended to organisations. Boswell (2008), for example, has argued that scientific knowledge plays a key role in legitimising the role of the European Commission in immigration policy, a field that is frequently inflicted with controversy. A similar observation was made by Bijker et al. (2009) in their study of the *Gezondheidsraad* (Health Council) in the Netherlands. They observed that the Council successfully utilised the authority of science to legitimise its advice to policy, which occurs – paradoxically, as they argue – despite the fact that contemporary society has become more critical of research and more aware of the limits of science (for example in relation to genetically modified food) (Weingart 1999). McNulty (2012) noted that aid organisations increasingly commission programme evaluation for the purpose of demonstrating compliance with expectations of accountability and transparency.

To be clear, the focus on strategic evidence use does not imply that scientific research is useless in informing policy-makers and in substantiating policy thinking in view of improving outcomes. However, it does raise the question of the motivation of policy-makers to use evidence and highlights the existence of considerations that have more to do with the nature of the policy process, the need to demonstrate accountability and the contested nature of decisions that affect the interests of policy actors than with conceptions of purely instrumental evidence use (Suchman 1995; Hansson 2006).

The case study of minimum volumes policy provides a pertinent example of evidence use in the face of conflicting interests played out in a corporatist system of health policy-making. The case also parallels controversies surrounding other decisions taken by the GBA, especially those to exclude or limit publicly funded services using health technology assessments

(HTA) (Perleth et al. 2009; Kieslich 2012). Such decisions can be highly controversial and pharmaceutical companies often take the GBA to court to challenge unfavourable outcomes. The threat of legal challenge requires the GBA to demonstrate the legitimacy of such decisions and it does so by reference to evidence reviews, commissioned from IQWIG, among other things. The role of HTA in legitimating potentially unpopular decisions about resource allocation (i.e. prioritisation, rationing) has also been critically discussed in relation to NICE, the National Institute of Health and Clinical Excellence in England (Syrett 2003; Littlejohns 2012), which is internationally recognised as a leader in this field. Yet while the GBA has a similar mandate and procedural arrangements are in place that are comparable to NICE, the legal framework and corporatist structures in which the GBA is embedded differ from the institutional context of NICE. NICE decisions are ultimately politically sanctioned by Government (not corporatist actors) and are less likely to attract legal redress due to differences in legal practice, while the GBA as a corporatist decision-maker is exposed to both influences of corporatist interests and opportunities for legal challenge (Syrett 2004; Gress et al. 2005; Francke and Hart 2008; Landwehr and Böhm 2011; Klingler et al. 2013).

METHODS

This case study is informed by documentary analysis and interviews. Documents include published protocols of parliamentary committees; published records of court decisions; selected articles from several broadsheet newspapers reporting on minimum volumes such as *Der Spiegel*, *Frankfurter Allgemeine Zeitung* and *Die Zeit* and from professional journals such as *Deutsches Ärzteblatt*; scientific reports published by IQWIG and by researchers commissioned to undertake evidence reviews; materials from websites such as policy documents relating to minimum volumes published by the GBA and by corporatist organisations, as well as press releases published by these organisations.

The documentary analysis has been supplemented by a number of interviews with key informants (n = 9), representing various types of policy-makers (government bureaucracy; corporatist organisations) and researchers. Interviewees were selected because of their knowledge of, and/or known involvement in, the process of developing minimum volumes policy. The roles of individual interviewees will not be identified in the following analysis to ensure the level of anonymity and confidentiality agreed at interview.

MINIMUM VOLUMES IN HOSPITAL: POLICY IDEA AND SCIENTIFIC EVIDENCE

Since the 1970s, health services research in the United States and elsewhere suggested that for certain services, typically complex surgery, hospitals that provided the service to a larger number of patients achieved better outcomes for patients (i.e. lower mortality and morbidity) than hospitals that provided the same service to a smaller number of patients (Luft et al. 1979). Interviewees suggested that studies published by Birkmeyer and colleagues in the 1990s and early 2000s were particularly influential in turning a statistically observed association of volume and outcomes into a policy idea (Birkmeyer et al. 1999, 2002, 2003; Finlayson et al. 2003). The idea also appealed to policy-makers as it resonated with the common sense notion that 'practice makes perfect'. Minimum volumes had already been ubiquitously used in medical training and accreditation, although they had not been used before to exclude hospitals from providing a service.

Regulating minimum volumes also fitted with the wider reform agenda for hospitals at the time. There were two concerns specifically: the perceived inefficiency and costliness of hospital care compared to other countries and emerging concerns about variation in the quality and outcomes of care. The first concern was to be addressed by the introduction of activity-based payments as the main method of funding hospitals (Busse and Blümel 2014). For their proponents, namely sickness funds, minimum volumes promised to speak to the second concern and to counter perceived risks to quality associated with the first.

However, despite being a policy idea inspired by scientific research, the scientific evidence base for operationalising the policy proved challenging. Evidence reviews suggested that there was a statistically significant relationship between higher volumes and improved outcomes for a number of complex surgical interventions such as pancreatic resection or oesophagectomy (Geraedts 2002; Rathmann and Windeler 2002; IQWiG 2005, 2008). These studies were typically observational (i.e. non-experimental) and were not considered as providing ultimate proof of causality. There were also limitations with regard to the data used in these studies, which typically relied on routinely collected information and were limited to certain populations or countries or groups of hospitals (e.g. in the US), raising questions about the transferability of their findings.

A further challenge was the difficulty of using studies indicating statistical correlations to support or set precise minimum volumes for specific procedures. Studies typically used definitions of 'high' and 'low' volumes of service provisions, but these were set by researchers and driven by data availability. In addition, most studies originated in the US, with studies using German data only emerging over time. But analyses of German data were also difficult to interpret and almost impossible to use to inform minimum volumes. For example, in 2006, IQWIG, the research institute associated with the GBA, published an analysis of data on volumes and outcomes of total knee replacement surgery, using two indicators of outcome quality (postsurgical mobility and infection) that produced conflicting findings (IQWiG 2006).

In sum, while there was scientific evidence to support the selection of services which could benefit from minimum volumes, there was limited evidence to guide the selection of the specific volumes to be set in these cases. This substantially reduced the potential for explicit "evidence based" decision-making when it came to setting volumes. Minimum volumes so far have not lent themselves to any straight forward translation of "evidence into policy". More importantly, however, they have been controversial from the outset, pitching against each other sickness funds as their proponents and hospitals as their vocal opposition. This conflict between payers and providers played out through all stages of the policy process with controversy surrounding the interpretation of the evidence often being at the centre of the argument. In addition, minimum volumes – as a regulatory policy – created winners and losers among hospitals, with smaller hospitals with fewer patients likely to lose out to large teaching hospitals. The opposition, represented in the German Hospital Association, was therefore not entirely unified, making it more difficult for hospitals to mount resistance.

DEVISING THE LEGISLATIVE FRAMEWORK

In 2001, the Federal Government – then composed of Social Democrats and the Green Party – brought a proposal for major reform of hospital funding before parliament. The proposal involved replacing the previous method of paying hospitals via budgets and per diems (payments per day of hospital stay) through a funding approach predominantly based on activity-based payments using diagnosis-related groups. The aim of this reform was to reduce perceived inefficiencies in hospital funding, reduce the length of stay of hospital inpatients, which were one of the longest in Europe, and to increase competition between hospitals. Minimum volumes were introduced on the back of this reform, as a counter measure to known risks to quality associated with activity-based funding as its proponents argued (*Interview*). They had the added attraction – especially for sickness funds and Social Democrats – of excluding hospitals with lower volumes from providing certain services, thus providing a lever for facilitating structural change in the (difficult to reform) hospital market.

Although the idea of regulating volumes of complex hospital services was inspired by research, scientific evidence, unsurprisingly, did not feature widely in the parliamentary discussion in which the legal framework for minimum volumes was developed. Instead, the procedural rules of parliamentary decision-making show a much clearer imprint on the resulting legislation, published as part of the 2002 Act on Case-Based Payment (*Fallpauschalengesetz*). In relation to minimum volumes, the 2002 Act stipulated that the relevant decision-making body of the self-administration (at that time the Hospital Committee and, from 2004, the GBA) should identify hospital services for which "the quality of outcomes particularly depended on the volume of services provided" and set minimum volumes for such services (Bundestag 2002b). The Act has since been integrated into Social Code Book V, now forming part of paragraph 137.

As the bill concerned hospital funding it directly touched on the legal responsibilities of the states and therefore required approval of both chambers of parliament. In the *Bundestag*, the bill was discussed in the Health Committee, which introduced a number of amendments including that minimum volumes should only be applied to 'planable' services (*planbar*), thus excluding urgent or emergency services. The Health Committee (composed of members of the *Bundestag* reflecting the proportionate representation of its constituent political parties) also requested transitional arrangements for hospitals that wanted to invest in expanding or creating new services, for example, by employing a new specialist (Bundestag 2001a). While seemingly reducing the scope of minimum volumes, the Health Committee also sharpened the bill by making minimum volumes binding on hospitals (instead of using them as guidelines as an earlier version suggested) and by preventing sickness funds from reimbursing services if hospitals continued to provide them in insufficient numbers. Taken together, the changes introduced by the Health Committee both suited the agenda of sickness funds and, to some extent, may have mollified hospitals by limiting minimum volumes to elective services only.

The states, represented in the *Bundesrat,* also made amendments to the bill as the documents of the Mediating Committee suggest. Specifically, the Committee (composed of members of the *Bundestag* and the *Bundesrat*) made provisions that allowed states to exempt individual hospitals from minimum volumes if they found access to services at risk within a given geographic area (Bundestag 2002a).

There is no indication in the documents examined that parliamentary committees concerned themselves with an interpretation of the scientific evidence available in support of minimum volumes. However, the resulting legislation, purposefully or unwittingly, included a clause where the specific wording lends itself to being interpreted as stipulating that specific minimum volumes had to be supported by scientific evidence. Specifically, the Act stated that "the quality of outcomes *particularly* depended on the volume of services provided" [emphasis added]. This clause had significant influence on how the law was subsequently interpreted and applied both by corporatist policy actors (i.e. the associations in favour and against, as well as the GBA as decision-making body) and by social courts involved in legal adjudication.

Setting Minimum Volumes: The Role of the Federal Joint Committee

With the passage of the Act, federal legislators mandated the self-administration to identify hospital services suitable for minimum volumes and to set volume thresholds. This task fell initially to the Hospital Committee (*Ausschuss Krankenhaus*), formed by the top associations of sickness funds, the German Hospital Association and the Medical Association (*Ärztekammer*), and, from 2004, to the newly formed GBA.

The legal mandate required associations of sickness funds and hospitals (with participation from a number of other organisations such as private health insurers) to jointly identify the 'catalogue of planable services' and to set minimum volumes for these services (MMV 2002). As constituents of the committee, both (groups of) associations brought their own positions and interests of their members to the negotiating table. Sickness funds, as noted above, were keen to establish minimum volumes as a policy instrument for quality assurance and structural change. The hospital association, in contrast, wanted to prevent their introduction and, as this had failed, to limit the number of services minimum volumes would apply to and keep volume thresholds low.

While unable to openly reject quality assurance as an objective, the main strategy of the hospital association was to highlight the risks to patients potentially arising from minimum volumes. These risks came in two flavours: The first argument was that minimum volumes would endanger access to care for patients by reducing the geographic coverage of services:

> In addition, the proposed bill suggests minimum volumes for hospitals. Yet the application of minimum volumes can exclude hospitals [from service provision] in an unjustified way, which would endanger access to services for patients. [DKG, Press release, 1 Feb 02]

A second line of argument was that minimum volumes were insufficiently supported by scientific evidence and were 'unfair' to low-volume hospitals that would produce good outcomes (*Interview*). Legislators had pre-empted the first line of argument by allowing state authorities to grant exemptions on a case-by-case basis on the grounds of geographic equity. However, the second argument – insufficient evidence – was more successful in challenging the appropriateness of minimum volumes and obstructing their implementation. This position has been maintained to this day in a slightly modified version, with the hospital association arguing that service volumes as surrogate parameter being less meaningful and therefore more likely to be unfair than indicators that measure quality directly (DKG 2014). While this is scientifically correct, it also raises the bar for regulation as it is not at all clear how other quality indicators would be operationalised to impact on hospitals' practice of service provision.

A first list of complex surgical procedures was agreed by the Hospital Committee in 2003, comprising liver transplants, kidney transplants, complex surgery of the oesophageal system and the pancreatic system, and stem cell transplantation. For these services, thresholds were set between 5 and 20 per hospital per year (liver transplantation 10; kidney translation 20; oesophageal surgery 5, pancreatic surgery 5, stem cell transplantation 10–14) (MMV 2002).

Interviewees commented that these procedures had been considered as relatively uncontroversial, as their share in service delivery and potential financial impact on hospitals was small and volume thresholds low (*Interview*). They were also reflective of the services analysed in existing studies (Geraedts 2002; Rathmann and Windeler 2002). The limited selection of services and the low thresholds thus suggest compromise between hospital and sickness fund associations on the lowest common denominator. In contrast, minimum volumes proposed by sickness funds (e.g. the *Verband der Angestellten-Krankenkassen*) had been much more ambitious, for example, for oesophageal and pancreatic surgery (both 10), coronary surgery (100), carotid surgery (20), percutaneous transluminal coronary angioplasty (150), breast cancer surgery (150) (Geraedts 2002).

In 2004, following the formation of the GBA, two further procedures were added to the list: total knee replacement and coronary surgery (BMGS 2004). However, no volumes were set at the time and coronary surgery – arguably a high volume service – would not be pursued any further. More controversially, in 2005, a threshold of 50 cases per hospital and year was set for total knee replacements (BMGS 2005). Neonatal services for babies with very low birth weight were added by the GBA in 2009 (GBA 2009). These two decisions involving services with high volumes (knee replacement) and high costs (neonatal care) proved highly contested and were both subsequently challenged in court by hospitals.

At the time, two 'evidence reports' – one commissioned by sickness funds and authored by Rathmann and Windeler (2002) and the other commissioned by the Federal Chamber of Physicians and authored by Geraedts (2002) – appeared to have influenced the selection of services for minimum volumes. Both reports were able to identify procedures such as complex surgery of oesophageal tumours for which evidence of a robust volume-outcome relationship existed. However, as these studies were observational and relied on routine data, their authors took care to mention that the evidence did not lend itself to suggesting volume thresholds. They also pointed out that studies did not identify the mechanisms, or factors, that would explain why higher volumes produced better outcomes. In other words, while these reviews established the problem and provided a rationale for action, they were unable to suggest specific solutions.

However, despite the known limitations of the evidence base, the 2003 agreement stipulated that future minimum volumes should be based on scientific evidence. Specifically, it stated that decisions should be taken based on 'epidemiological and empirical knowledge' and applied in 'a transparent and rule-based process' (MMV 2002: 1). Not only should future minimum volumes require evidence of a causal relationship between volume and outcomes, they also required proof that improved outcomes were *predominantly* caused by higher volumes (*'im überwiegenden Teil'*). Thus the 2003 agreement suggested that minimum volumes should only be set if volume was proven to be the decisive factor for variation in outcomes. This wording echoed similar terminology in the law ('*in besonderem Maße*') but further raised the bar as to which types of evidence were regarded sufficient. However, evidence of volume being more influential than other factors was difficult to come by for practical reasons (i.e. such studies did not exist) and scientific reasons (i.e. volume is a proxy for other factors thus can never be decisive).

Unsurprisingly, this move towards evidence-based medicine in justifying minimum volumes was celebrated by the hospital association:

> Paragraph 3 of the agreement includes a procedural rule that stipulates that the setting of minimum volumes for certain services require an evidence-based process and scientific evaluation. [DKV, 4 Dec 03]

In 2004, having replaced the Hospital Committee, the GBA asked its newly created research institute, IQWiG, to examine the evidence of a volume-outcome relationship and to identify thresholds for total knee replacement (IQWiG 2005). Published in 2005, the IQWiG report noted that a volume-outcome relationship was plausible, but could not be proven in the absence of experimental studies (IQWiG 2005). In addition, the analysis of hospital data on volumes and outcomes for total knee replacement (using the outcome measures 'post-surgical mobility' and 'infection after surgery') resulted in conflicting findings, with one indicator showing a decline in desired outcomes at higher volumes and the other showing steady improvement. Individually and jointly the analyses of these indicators did not indicate that there is an ideal volume threshold. A later report by IQWiG relating to the treatment of very premature babies with very low birth weight also concluded that a causal relationship between volume and outcomes was likely, but could not be regarded as ultimately proven due to the absence of experimental studies (IQWiG 2008).

Since its inception the GBA has been committed to stringent evidence use, prompted by controversies over the reimbursement of pharmaceuticals and medical procedures, often involving legal action from manufacturers. There has also been a drive to professionalise procedures with several documents specifying its by-laws and code of practice. There was a notable effort to apply similarly robust approaches to decisions on minimum volumes, resulting in the commissioning of reviews and additional data analyses prepared by IQWiG. In commissioning these studies, the GBA explicitly followed established best practice, including the publication of protocols and peer review. In compliance with its by-laws, the GBA provided explicit rationales for its decisions, made this information publicly available and gave due consideration to reports commissioned from its research institute (GBA 2008).

Yet despite this emphasis on procedural robustness, the GBA found itself in a position in which it was impossible to base minimum volume decisions on evidence alone. This happened because the scientific evidence in support of specific threshold was inconclusive. In addition, being a membership organisation, the GBA continued to be exposed to the partisan interests of its member organisations, in one instance rejecting a study brought in by the hospital association which aimed to demonstrate that a volume-outcome relationship was inexistent (GBA 2010). There was thus substantial tension between two procedural rules, those set out in by-laws which aim at ensuring transparency and due process, and those associated with the corporatist nature of the GBA and the practice of negotiating consensus between the organised interests in health care. In the end, decisions about minimum volumes were taken by majority vote, which overruled the resistance of the hospital association. Yet this did not end the controversy.

ADJUDICATION BY THE SOCIAL COURTS

Following the introduction of minimum volumes for total knee replacement at a level of 50 per hospital and year and of increasing existing volumes for very premature babies from 14 to 30 (GBA 2013), several hospitals took legal action against sickness funds which had refused to pay for services delivered at lower numbers than required. Both cases led to a judicial review of the GBA decisions at state level (the Social Court of Berlin-Brandenburg, here referred to as 'state court'), and, subsequently, at federal level (by the Federal Social Court, here the 'federal court').

Three questions were considered in the courts specifically: (1). Whether the GBA was entitled to set minimum volumes that are binding on hospitals; (2). whether the selection of services to apply minimum volumes to was in compliance with the law (i.e. SGB 5), especially whether these services were 'planable' (in the case of services for preterm babies) and whether there was sufficient evidence of a 'particular' relationship between volume and outcome; and (3). whether specific minimum volumes set had been sufficiently justified by the GBA, including by recourse to scientific evidence.

On the first question, the state and federal courts upheld consistently that the GBA was entitled and mandated by parliament to set binding minimum volumes; however, the courts emphasised that, in compliance with German administrative law, the GBA had to explain and justify such decisions (BSG 2012a, b).

On the second question, the federal court ruled that services are legitimately selected if they are 'planable' in the sense that they can be accessed without posing additional risks to patients, arising, for example, from longer journeys to (fewer) hospitals. In relation to care for very premature babies, the court argued, referencing national and international studies, that the benefits for mothers-to-be outweighed the risks associated with longer travel (BSG 2012a: para 43). The court thus rejected an interpretation of 'planable' as 'elective' or 'predictable', as both terms would not consider the balance of risks and benefits to patients (BSG 2012a: para 30).

The courts also referred to research to clarify the meaning of the law with regard to the 'particular' causal relationship between volumes and outcomes required by law to justify specific minimum volumes. In 2011, the state court ruled that a causal relationship could only be regarded as 'particular' if 'controlled studies' suggested a statistical relationship (LSG 2011: para 87). The state court thus aligned the wording of the law with the concept of the 'hierarchy of evidence' used in evidence-based medicine, which considers RCTs as the strongest research design to establish claims of causality.

This ruling was revised by the federal court in 2012 and confirmed in subsequent decisions in 2014 and 2015. The federal court argued that the law should not be interpreted as giving preference to particularly types of studies, especially since in the case of minimum volumes RCTs were neither practical nor ethical. Evidence from scientific studies would suffice if a causal relationship was 'probable and plausible' (BSG 2012b: para 31). However, such decisions would require additional support in the form of 'medical experience' (*medizinische Erfahrungssätze*) (BSG 2012b: 39). Such medical experience is often used in court decisions by inviting expert witnesses (*Sachverständige*), although in this case the courts largely relied on written statements from the GBA in justification if its position.

The third question discussed by the courts was whether specific minimum volumes had been sufficiently explained and justified by the GBA. The review of such justifications drew heavily on scientific evidence, although courts came to different conclusions about the level of justification needed for minimum volumes to be considered legal. For the state court in 2011, evidence was insufficient in the absence of experimental studies, which meant that the minimum volumes in question were unjustified (LSG 2011). Rejecting this ruling, the federal court argued – in line with its earlier reasoning – that minimum volumes were sufficiently justified if they were likely to improve outcomes, if the statistical association would be supported by 'medical experience' and if potential risks arising from minimum volumes (e.g. longer distances) would be outweighed by the potential benefits (BSG 2012a, 2014).

This weighing of risks and benefits led the federal court to come to different conclusions when considering specific minimum volumes. It argued that minimum volumes of 14 cases of very preterm babies per year were justified noting that 14 cases (roughly one per month) were sufficient to require the presence of a specialist team in a hospital. The existence of such a team would make quality improvements plausible. In a similar vein, it argued that 50 total knee replacements (roughly one per week on average) would be sufficient to require the hospital to employ a specialist team (BSG 2012a, 2014).

Using the same rationale, the federal court rejected minimum volumes of 30 per year for very preterm babies on the grounds that the higher threshold would increase the risks to those babies by excluding hospitals with lower volumes (but potentially providing good quality services) without necessarily increasing the benefits (BSG 2012b: para 60–61). It specifically cited four studies in support of this suggestion, one of which had been included in a systematic review (i.e. by IQWiG) and another one had been rejected by the GBA in an earlier version and was co-funded by the hospital association (GBA 2010; Kutschmann et al. 2012). While these studies made valid points about the limited ability of minimum volumes to separate high from low performing hospitals entirely accurately, the ruling gave prominence to a few selected studies while disregarding all the others included in previous scientific reviews.

In conclusion, the analysis of court decisions suggests that scientific evidence was of relevance to the legal adjudication on minimum volumes to establish whether specific minimum volumes set by the GBA were sufficiently justified in the eyes of the law. However, the decision itself was not based on evidence but on principles of plausibility and proportionality established in legal practice, which were then supported by research. Key to establishing conformity with the law was that the setting of minimum volumes was demonstrably proven to have been deliberated, with consideration given to the available evidence, and that a justification was provided that could be reviewed in court.

DISCUSSION AND CONCLUSION

This chapter has examined the development of minimum volume policy as a case study of health policy making in Germany. It specifically analysed the policy process and the way in which policy decisions were supported by evidence. It has argued that evidence use was mostly strategic: corporatist actors such as the hospital association and sickness funds commissioned research to support their aims; the hospital association consistently promoted evidence use (specifically the 'highest' level of evidence such as RCTs, which for minimum volumes does not exist) as a cornerstone of decisions on specific minimum volumes; it also brought in its own, i.e. co-funded, studies to underline its position that minimum volumes do not make a meaningful contribution to quality assurance.

The formation of the GBA and IQWiG in 2004 has changed the rules of the argumentative game, with new procedures developed for, and applied to, decision-making and scientific evidence use. Decision-making had previously been dominated by the consensual arrangements characteristic of corporatism. Consensual arrangements have been maintained in the GBA to some extent, however, decisions are eventually taken by majority vote, which means that resistance by providers can be overcome provided there is a majority. Decision-making procedures have become more rule-based, for example as they relate to commissioning evidence reviews from the IQWIG and considering its findings. This suggests that scientific evidence has become a substantial aspect of the GBA's approach to legitimising its decisions in relation to minimum volumes. This chimes with findings from Boswell (2008), as well as Bijker et al. (2009), which describe the transfer of scientific authority to decision-making bodies helping them to legitimise their actions. Similar observations have been made in relation to decisions involving HTA where the legislator has recently tightened the framework for decisions for inpatient services preventing the GBA to exclude services in the absence of evidence. New hospital services have to be proven to be either less effective than existing treatments or harmful, thus setting a high bar to evidentiary support for decisions about service exclusions (Olberg et al. 2014).

Still, in relation to minimum volumes the analysis also echoes findings that emphasise the negotiated nature of decisions (Etgeton 2009), suggesting that policy actors who are constituent members of the GBA engage in strategic uses of evidence to support their claims and promote their interests. Corporatist structures have changed and become more pluralist, adversarial and less consensus oriented. While some have argued that the GBA is particularly well placed for taking unpopular decisions in contested policy fields such as service exclusions from the public benefits package (Gerlinger 2010), the present state of affairs suggests that such decisions often end up in court. Courts then weigh the scientific evidence provided in support of a decision to establish whether the GBA has provided sufficient justification, although cognisant (perhaps increasingly so) of the limits of such evidence. This analysis suggests however that substantive disagreements between different organised interests do not disappear by evoking the authority of scientific evidence. Evidence use as 'technocratic fix' is unlikely to solve the legitimacy problems of organisations charged with unpopular decisions (Syrett 2003). Decisions that directly affect the interests of policy actors, perhaps especially so if these have financial implications and impact on notions of professional autonomy, are likely to remain contested and have a fair chance to require legal adjudication. The GBA is routinely taken to court by pharmaceutical producers (and sometimes patients) contesting decisions to exclude medicinal products from public reimbursement, which is a well-trodden (though not necessarily successful) avenue given that access to legal review is easy in the German legal system. In this case here, smaller hospitals are particularly likely to be affected by minimum volumes and while the hospital association opposed the policy almost throughout (although there are signs of partial acceptance following repeated confirmation by the judiciary (DKG 2014)) hospitals affected by the policy have found their interests directly at stake and have sought legal redress individually.

The policy process analysed here arguably does not tell the full story of minimum volumes, as it focuses on three specific stages of decision-making while largely ignoring the dynamics of agenda-setting prior to the parliamentary debate, and the actual impact of minimum volumes in practice. There is now clear evidence that minimum volume regulation is widely ignored by hospitals and sickness funds are incapable of retrieving funding from hospitals if services turn out to have been delivered in volumes below the threshold (de Cruppé et al. 2014; Peschke et al. 2014).

Court decisions also have tended to directly affect how the GBA went about making decisions, with some noting that the first court cases led to more attention given to future evidentiary support for decisions. It also led to the GBA ceasing to introduce further minimum volumes. Meanwhile, sickness funds have asked parliament to change the wording of the law to reduce the requirement on evidentiary support for minimum volumes

(Leber 2014). In December 2015, a new law (the *Act to Reform the Structures of Hospital Provision*, KHSG) removed the phrase 'in besonderem Maße' (i.e. the *particular* relationship of volume and outcome) from the SGB 5 to make specific minimum volumes more defensible in court and introduce a process that would make it easier for sickness funds to withhold funding from hospitals for services under the threshold. Whether this will increase the number of minimum volumes introduced by the GBA in future and, indeed, further changes the balance between payers and providers in the still corporatist system of health policy making in Germany remains to be seen.

The analysis above has shown that various forms of strategic evidence use dominate the example of minimum volume policy in Germany. While it is clear that strategic use of evidence does not entirely preclude notions of 'evidence-based policy' – as evidence can also have a substantive impact on decisions – this analysis suggests that expectations of 'instrumental' evidence use are likely to be disappointed. Changes in corporatist decision-making, namely the formation of the GBA, have brought about new opportunities for evidence use, necessitated by the GBA's need to legitimise its decisions, including in court. But this has not reduced the potential for contestation or has fully established the idea of instrumental (i.e. objective) evidence use.

These findings hint at the contextual nature of evidence use in policy-making, which is shaped by the specific institutional arrangements of health care governance and the wider political system that influence the motivation of policy actors and organisations to use evidence to legitimise decisions. While the case of minimum volumes has shown that evidentiary support is necessary for such GBA decisions, evidence was not the only, or indeed most relevant, source of legitimacy, as legitimation is also derived from parliamentary law-making, corporatist governance and legal adjudication by the judiciary.

REFERENCES

Bandelow, N. 2004. Akteure und Interessen in der Gesundheitspolitik: Vom Korporatismus zum Pluralismus? *Politische Bildung* 37 (1): 49–63.
———. 2009. Health governance in the aftermath of traditional corporatism: One small step for the legislator, one giant leap for the subsystem? *German Policy Studies* 5 (1): 43–63.
Bijker, W.E., R. Bal, and R. Hendriks. 2009. *The paradox of scientific authority. The role of scientific advice in democracies*. Cambridge, MA: MIT Press.

Birkmeyer, J.D., S.R. Finlayson, A.N. Tosteson, S.M. Sharp, A.L. Warshaw, and E.S. Fisher. 1999. Effect of hospital volume on in-hospital mortality with pancreaticoduodenectomy. *Surgery* 125 (3): 250–256.
Birkmeyer, J.D., A.E. Siewers, E.V. Finlayson, T.A. Stukel, F.L. Lucas, I. Batista, H.G. Welch, and D.E. Wennberg. 2002. Hospital volume and surgical mortality in the United States. *New England Journal of Medicine* 346 (15): 1128–1137.
Birkmeyer, J.D., T.A. Stukel, A.E. Siewers, P.P. Goodney, D.E. Wennberg, and F.L. Lucas. 2003. Surgeon volume and operative mortality in the United States. *New England Journal of Medicine* 349 (22): 2117–2127.
Blum, S., and K. Schubert, eds. 2013. *Policy analysis in Germany*. Bristol: Policy Press.
BMGS. 2004. Beschluss des Gemeinsamen Bundesausschusses nach § 91 Abs. 7 des Fünften Buches Sozialgesetzbuch (SGB V) zur Aufnahme in den Mindestmengenkatalog nach § 137 Abs. 1 Satz 3 Nr. 3 SGB V vom 21. September 2004. Berlin, Bundesministerium für Gesundheit und Soziale Sicherung.
———. 2005. Bekanntmachung eines Beschlusses des Gemeinsamen Bundesausschusses nach § 91 Abs. 7 des Fünften Buches Sozialgesetzbuch (SGB V) zur Festlegung einer Mindestmenge nach § 137 Abs. 1 Satz 3 SGB V vom 16. August 2005. Berlin, Bundesministerium für Gesundheit und Soziale Sicherung.
Boswell, C. 2008. The political functions of expert knowledge: Knowledge and legitimation in European Union immigration policy. *Journal of European Public Policy* 15 (4): 471–488.
BSG. 2012a. Urteil vom 12 September, B 3 KR 10/12 R. Kassel, Bundessozialgericht.
———. 2012b. Urteil vom 18 Dezember, B 1 KR 34/12 R. Kassel, Bundessozialgericht.
———. 2014. Urteil vom 14 Oktober 2014, B 1 KR 33/13 R. Kassel, Bundessozialgericht.
Bundestag. 2001a. Bericht des Ausschusses für Gesundheit, 14. Wahlperiode, Drucksache 14/7862. Berlin, Deutscher Bundestag.
———. 2001b. Beschlussempfehlung des Ausschusses für Gesundheit, 14. Wahlperiode, Drucksache 14/7824. Berlin, Deutscher Bundestag.
———. 2002a. Beschlussempfehlung des Vermittlungsausschusses zu dem Gesetz zur Einführung des diagnose-orientierten Fallpauschalensystems für Krankenhäuser (Fallpauschalengesetz – FPG), 14. Wahlperiode, Drucksache 14/8362. Berlin, Deutscher Bundestag.
———. 2002b. Gesetz zur Einführung des diagnose-orientierten Fallpauschalensystems für Krankenhäuser (Fallpauschalengesetz – FPG). *Bundesgesetzblatt* 1: 1412–1438.
Busse, R., and M. Blümel. 2014. Germany: Health system review. *Health Systems in Transition* 10 (2): 1–296.

de Cruppé, W., M. Malik, and M. Geraedts. 2014. Umsetzung der Mindestmengenvorgaben: Analyse der Krankenhausqualitätsberichte. *Deutsches Ärzteblatt* 111 (33–34): 549–555.

DKG. 2014. *Positionen der Deutschen Krankenhausgesellschaft zur Weiterentwicklung der Qualitätssicherung und der Patientensicherheit*. Berlin: Deutsche Krankenhausgesellschaft.

Etgeton, S. 2009. Patientenbeteiligung in den Strukturen des Gemeinsamen Bundesausschusses. *Bundesgesundheitsblatt-Gesundheitsforschung-Gesundheitsschutz* 52 (1): 104–110.

Finlayson, E.V., P.P. Goodney, and J.D. Birkmeyer. 2003. Hospital volume and operative mortality in cancer surgery: A national study. *Archives of Surgery* 138 (7): 721–725.

Francke, R., and D. Hart. 2008. Einführung in die rechtlichen Aspekte bei HTAs. *Zeitschrift fuer Evidenz, Fortbildung und Qualität im Gesundheitswesen* 102: 63–68.

GBA. 2008. Verfahrensordnung des Gemeinsamen Bundesausschusses (in its version of January 2014). Berlin: Gemeinsamer Bundesausschuss.

———. 2009. Bekanntmachung eines Beschlusses des Gemeinsamen Bundesausschusses zur Versorgung von Früh- und Neugeborenen vom 20. Bundesanzeiger 195: 4450.

———. 2010. Tragende Gründe zum Beschluss des Gemeinsamen Bundesausschusses über eine Änderung der Anlage 1 der Mindestmengevereinbarung: Mindestmengen bei Früh- und Neugeborenen vom 17. Juni. Berlin: Gemeinsamer Bundesausschuss.

———. 2013. *Geschaeftsbericht 2012*. Berlin: Gemeinsamer Bundesausschuss.

Geraedts, M. 2002. Evidenz zur Ableitung von Mindestmengen in der Medizin. Gutachten im Auftrag der Bundesärztekammer. Düsseldorf, Heinrich-Heine-Universität.

Gerlinger, T. 2010. Health care reform in Germany. *German Policy Studies* 6 (1): 107–142.

Greenhalgh, T., and J. Russell. 2007. Reframing evidence synthesis as rhetorical action in the policy making drama. *Politiques de Santé* 1: 34–42.

Gress, S., D. Niebuhr, H. Rothgang, and J. Wasem. 2005. Criteria and procedures for determining benefits packages in health care. A comparative perspective. *Health Policy* 73: 78–91.

Hansson, F. 2006. Organizational use of evaluations: Governance and control in research evaluation. *Evaluation* 12 (2): 159–178.

Hind, D. 2007. *The threat to reason: How the enlightenment was hijacked and how we can reclaim it*. London: Verso.

IQWiG. 2005. Entwicklung und Anwendung von Modellen zur Berechnung von Schwellenwerten bei Mindestmengen für Knie-Totalendoprothese. Abschlussbericht. Cologne: Institut für Qualität und Wirtschaftlichkeit im Gesundheitswesen.

———. 2006. Entwicklung und Erstellung eines Prognosemodells zur Ermittlung der Auswirkungen von Schwellenwerten auf die Versorgung. Abschlussbericht. Cologne: Institut für Qualität und Wirtschaftlichkeit im Gesundheitswesen.

———. 2008. Zusammenhang zwischen Leistungsmenge und Ergebnis bei der Versorung von Früh- und Neugeborenen mit sehr geringem Geburtsgewicht. Abschlussbericht. Cologne, Institut für Qualität und Wirtschaftlichkeit im Gesundheitswesen.

———. 2015. Aufgaben und Ziele des IQWiG. https://www.iqwig.de/de/ueber-uns/aufgaben-und-ziele.2946.html. Accessed 14 Jan 2015.

Jun, U., and K. Grabow. 2008. *Mehr Expertise in der deutschen Politik? Zur Übertragbarkeit des "Evidence-based policy approach"*. Bertelsmann Stiftung: Gütersloh.

Kieslich, K. 2012. Social values and health priority setting in Germany. *Journal of Health Organization and Management* 26 (3): 374–383.

Klingler, C., S.M. Shah, A.J. Barron, and J.S. Wright. 2013. Regulatory space and the contextual mediation of common functional pressures: Analyzing the factors that led to the German Efficiency Frontier approach. *Health Policy* 109: 270–280.

Kloten, N. 2006. Wissenschaftliche Beratung der Politik: Befund und Auftrag. Politikberatung in Deutschland. Heidelberger Akademie der Wissenschaften. Wiesbaden, VS Verlag für Sozialwissenschaften: 123–145.

Knieps, F. 2009. Evidence based health policy oder wissenschaftlich verbrämter Lobbyismus – Die Verwertung wissenschaftlicher Erkenntnisse in der Gesundheitspolitik. *Zeitschrift für Evidenz, Fortbildung und Qualität im Gesundheitswesen* 103 (5): 273–280.

Kutschmann, M., S. Bungard, J. Kötting, A. Trümner, C. Fusch, and C. Veit. 2012. Versorgung von Frühgeborenen mit einem Geburtsgewicht unter 1 250 g. *Deutsches Ärzteblatt* 109 (31–32): 519–528.

Landwehr, C., and K. Böhm. 2011. Delegation and institutional design in healthcare rationing. *Governance: An International Journal of Policy, Administration, and Institutions* 24 (4): 665–688.

Leber, W.-D. 2014. Mindestmengen. AQUA-Tagung „Qualität kennt keine Grenzen", Göttingen, May 14. http://tagung-2014.sqg.de/2014/ppt/P4-1-fol_G%C3%B6ttingen_2014_05_14_AQUA_Mindestmengen_Dr%20Leber_final.pdf. Accessed 17 Jan 2015.

Lehmbruch, G. 1988. Der Neokorporatismus der Bundesrepublik im internationalen Vergleich und die „Konzertierte Aktion im Gesundheitswesen ". Neokorporatismus und Gesundheitswesen. G. Gäfgen. Baden-Baden, Nomos: 11–32.

Lijphart, A., and M. Crepaz. 1991. Corporatism and consensus democracy in eighteen countries: Conceptual and empirical linkages. *British Journal of Political Science* 21 (2): 235–246.

Littlejohns, P. 2012. Social values and health priority setting in England: 'values' based decision making. *Journal of Health Organization and Management* 26 (3): 363–371.

LSG. 2011. Urteil vom 17. August 2011, L 7 KA 77/08 KL. Potsdam, Landessozialgericht Berlin-Brandenburg.
Luft, H.S., J.P. Bunker, and A.C. Enthoven. 1979. Should operations be regionalized? The empirical relation between surgical volume and mortality. *The New England Journal of Medicine* 301 (25): 1364–1369.
Majone, G. 1989. *Evidence, argument, and persuasion in the policy process.* Yale: Yale University Press.
Marmot, M.G. 2004. Evidence based policy or policy based evidence? Willingness to take action influences the view of the evidence – Look at alcohol. *BMJ* 328: 906–907.
Mayntz, R. 2009. Speaking truth to power: Leitlinien für die Regelung wissenschaftlicher Politikberatung. *Zeitschrift fuer Public Policy, Recht und Management* 1: 5–16.
McNulty, J. 2012. Symbolic uses of evaluation in the international aid sector: Arguments for critical reflection. *Evidence & Policy: A Journal of Research, Debate and Practice* 8 (4): 495–509.
MMV. 2002. Vereinbarung gemäss Paragraph 137 Abs. 1 Satz 3 Nr. 3 SGB 5 – Mindestmengenvereinbarung.
Olberg, B., M. Perleth, and R. Busse. 2014. The new regulation to investigate potentially beneficial diagnostic and therapeutic methods in Germany: Up to international standard? *Health Policy* 117: 135–145.
Perleth, M., B. Gibis, and B. Goehlen. 2009. A short history of health technology assessment in Germany. *International Journal of Technology Assessment in Health Care* 25 (Suppl 1): 112–119.
Peschke, D., U. Nimptsch, and T. Mansky. 2014. Umsetzung der Mindestmengenvorgaben: Analyse der DRG-Daten. *Deutsches Ärzteblatt* 111 (33-34): 556–563.
Rathmann, W., and J. Windeler. 2002. Zusammenhang zwischen Behandlungsmenge und Behandlungsqualität. Evidenzbericht. Essen: Medizinischer Dienst der Spitzenverbände der Krankenkassen.
Renn, O. 1995. Style of using scientific expertise: A comparative framework. *Science and Public Policy* 22 (3): 147–156.
Siefken, S.T. 2007. *Expertenkommissionen im politischen Prozess. Eine Bilanz zur rot-grünen Bundesregierung 1998–2005.* Wiesbaden: VS Verlag für Sozialwissenschaften.
Strueck, C. 2013. Public interest groups and policy analysis: A push for evidence-based policy-making? In *Policy analysis in Germany*, ed. S. Blum and K. Schubert, 217–230. Bristol: Policy Press.
Suchman, M.C. 1995. Managing legitimacy: Strategic and institutional approaches. *Academy of Management Review* 20 (3): 571–610.

Syrett, K. 2003. A technocratic fix to the 'legitimacy problem'? The Blair Government and health care rationing in the United Kingdom. *Journal of Health Politics, Policy and Law* 28 (4): 715–746.
———. 2004. Impotence or importance? Judicial review in an era of explicit NHS rationing. *Modern Law Review* 67 (2): 289–321.
Tsebelis, G. 2011. *Veto players: How political institutions work*. Princeton: Princeton University Press.
Weingart, P. 1999. Scientific expertise and political accountability: Paradoxes of sciences in politics. *Science and Public Policy* 26 (3): 151–161.
Weiss, C.H. 1979. The many meanings of research utilization. *Public Administration Review* 39 (5): 426–431.

Open Access   This chapter is licensed under the terms of the Creative Commons Attribution 4.0 International License (http://creativecommons.org/licenses/by/4.0/), which permits use, sharing, adaptation, distribution and reproduction in any medium or format, as long as you give appropriate credit to the original author(s) and the source, provide a link to the Creative Commons license and indicate if changes were made.

The images or other third party material in this chapter are included in the chapter's Creative Commons license, unless indicated otherwise in a credit line to the material. If material is not included in the chapter's Creative Commons license and your intended use is not permitted by statutory regulation or exceeds the permitted use, you will need to obtain permission directly from the copyright holder.

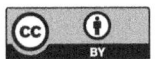

CHAPTER 7

Electronic Cigarettes Regulation in the UK: A Case Study in Evidence Informed Policy Making

Benjamin Hawkins

INTRODUCTION

Electronic cigarettes (e-cigarettes) are hand-held, battery-operated devices, in which liquid nicotine is vapourised and inhaled by the user. E-cigarettes vary greatly in form and appearance, with some products (known as 'cigalikes') closely resembling conventional cigarettes in shape and appearance. Larger, refillable devices (known as 'eGos' or 'mods') bear little visual similarity to tobacco products (Zhu et al. 2014; Grana et al. 2014a). The latter offer the possibility for users to vary rates of nicotine delivery through adjustable settings, customisation and the concentration of nicotine solution ('e-liquid') used. Globally, transnational tobacco corporations (TTCs) have aggressively entered the sector through a series of mergers and acquisitions (Manning 2013; Richtel 2013; McNeill and Munafò 2013; Tobacco Tactics 2014a) and the once highly disparate e-cigarette market is rapidly

B. Hawkins (✉)
London School of Hygiene and Tropical Medicine, London, UK
e-mail: ben.hawkins@lshtm.ac.uk

© The Author(s) 2018
J. Parkhurst et al. (eds.), *Evidence Use in Health Policy Making*,
International Series on Public Policy,
https://doi.org/10.1007/978-3-319-93467-9_7

consolidating around a small number of producers, linked to TTCs (Smithers 2014; Thesing 2014).

Studies indicate that use of e-cigarettes doubled in Europe and North America between 2008 and 2012 (Grana et al. 2014a). The rapid expansion in the use and marketing of these products raised a number of regulatory issues including their classification (as consumer products or medical devices), and thus the ways in which they can be sold and marketed, and restrictions on their purchase (age limits and outlet types) and use (in public places) (World Health Organization 2014). As the popularity and promotion of e-cigarettes grew, national governments and the European Union (EU) sought to put in place effective rules governing their sale, use and marketing, which balance the potential benefits of e-cigarettes (primarily for existing smokers who may use them as quit aids) against the need to protect consumers and the wider public's health.

Policy decisions such as how to regulate e-cigarettes require responsible agencies to evaluate the likely impact and potential risks of novel products, through engagement with the relevant bodies of evidence. In the case of e-cigarettes, this process was complicated by the limited evidence base on the health effects of e-cigarettes in real world conditions or their patterns of use and the significant divisions which have emerged within the tobacco control and public health communities regarding e-cigarettes (cf. Etter 2013; Chapman 2013; Chapman et al. 2017; McNeill et al. 2015a; McKee and Capewell 2015a). Those in favour on e-cigarettes emphasise their potential usefulness as smoking cessations tools, and emphasise that e-cigarettes offer a market oriented and demand led solution to smoking. Consequently they support non–interventionist regulatory frameworks which facilitate the development of the product category and their appeal to smokers. Against this, those concerned about the potentially negative externalities of e-cigarettes for population level health have advocated policy makers adopt the precautionary principle and more robust controls on the sale, marketing and use of e-cigarettes. This schism has seen two separate letters sent to WHO Director-General, Margaret Chan, setting out the potential benefits and dangers of e-cigarettes respectively, and advocating very different regulatory approaches to the products (Abrams et al. 2014; Aktan et al. 2014; Gartner and Malone 2014). In the UK, a key market for the e-cigarette category and the policy debate on their regulation, the division between public health advocates in favour of or opposed to e-cigarettes came to the fore following publication of a Public Health England Report (McNeill et al. 2015a, b) endorsing the positive health effects of e-cigarettes and subsequent criticisms from other public health actors (McKee and Capewell 2015a, b; Lancet 2015).

It is widely accepted that a highly unified advocacy and NGO network, coalescing around a shared policy agenda, has played a key role in delivering advances in tobacco control in recent decades (Gneiting 2015; Wipfli 2015). E-cigarettes can thus be seen as a disruptive force in the field of tobacco policy, problematizing accepted norms of evidence use in decision making and dividing the expert community to which the government had previously been able to turn for clear, coherent guidance in this area.

The issue of e-cigarettes thus offers a highly pertinent case through which to study the process of evidence-use in policy making. Furthermore, the UK is a particularly useful context in which to examine evidence use in e-cigarette debates for four main reasons. First, the UK has a long-standing, and deeply embedded, culture of evidence use in policy making dating back at least to the New Labour Government (Parsons 2002), which has seen norms of evidence use institutionalised in bodies such as the National Institute of Health and Care Excellence (NICE). Second, the idea that health policy should be informed by research evidence is widely accepted, both within policy making circles and amongst the wider public (Cairney and Studlar 2014; Smith 2013). This is reflected in the strong rhetorical commitment to the goal of 'evidence-based' policy amongst both decision-makers and policy advocates in relation to e-cigarettes. Third, the UK has a strong record on tobacco control and some of the most advanced tobacco control policies in the world (ASH 2007). As elsewhere, this was achieved to a significant extent by the successful advocacy of a well organised and unified public health community, which has been divided by the issue of e-cigarettes. Finally, the UK has been the site of some of the most vehement policy debates on e-cigarettes globally and some of the most bitter disagreements over the nature of the policy challenge posed by e-cigarettes and the guidance offered by the existing research evidence.

E-Cigarette Regulation in the UK

In EU member-states, many aspects of e-cigarette regulation are decided collectively at the European level. The 2014 Tobacco Products Directive (TPD) which governs the sale and marketing of e-cigarettes in the UK, takes a dual approach in which devices meeting certain criteria (such as the concentration of nicotine solution they contain) may be sold as tobacco products under the auspices of the Directive, whilst others must be licenced as medical devices by the designated national authorities, such as the UK Medicines and Healthcare Products Regulatory Agency (MHRA). This classification determines how their sale, use and marketing are regulated, with only medical devices able to make health claims. National governments remain responsible for other areas of e-cigarette policy without cross border effects including minimum purchase ages for e-cigarettes and rules relating to their use in public places. Public Health England have played a prominent role in discussions about the regulation of e-cigarettes (Bauld et al. 2014; Dockrell et al. 2013; McNeill et al. 2015a), including the issue of public use which, following the implementation of the TPD has emerged as a key point of contention between actors (Chapman et al. 2017; Bauld et al. 2016).

Issue Framing and Evidence Informed Policy

As is argued throughout the current volume, recent contributions to the study of evidence-informed policy making problematise both our understanding of research evidence and evidence use in the policy process, recognising that that there can be multiple bodies of evidence of relevance to a given policy issue, where multiple (and perhaps mutually exclusive) concerns and policy priorities are at stake in the context of finite governmental resources available to address them. The issue of policy framing is, therefore, key to the analysis of the development of e-cigarette policy debates and the role of evidence within these (Van Hulst and Yanow 2016; Koon et al. 2016). The way policy controversies are framed – the specific understanding of what the issue at stake is – will lead different, relevant bodies of evidence to be foregrounded in debates. Equally, frame sponsors – policy advocates promoting particular understanding of policy issues – pursue particular policy agendas and will point to different bodies of evidence as an argumentative too to support their position (Majone 1993).

Disagreements over what the issue is cannot be decided by recourse to evidence, since interlocutors will not agree on what the 'right' issue framing (and thus the relevant body of evidence) is. However, policy actors often misapprehend that they are engaged, not in debates about the facts of the issue, but in a debate about what this issue itself is; how it is defined and which account of that issue prevails (Stone 1989; Bacchi 2009). The process of issue framing and agenda setting is highly political and involves conflicts between competing values, priorities and ideologies in the context of finite resources. In some cases, the competing values at stake in policy debates may be mutually exclusive and come into direct conflict (e.g. concerns over freedoms and civil liberties versus security). At other times, governments may have to decide to prioritise certain issues and outcomes over others, and this may be the result of successful discursive strategies by frame sponsors including the provision of evidence to support their claims.

Crucially, policy actors are often unable to see that they and their opponents are talking about fundamentally different things – or understand the policy problem to be something fundamentally different – even where they address what seems to be the 'same' issue through the 'same' vocabulary. As Charles Taylor (1971) comments, arguments over common meanings are often the basis of the most vehement political disputes. Making explicit and recognising the particular perspectives from which we see certain issues – our own biases and preferences that dictate what the issue *is* for us – has been identified as an essential step in overcoming protracted political controversies in a process of 'frame reflection' (Rein and Schön 1994).

Whilst intractable policy disputes of this kind cannot be resolved by recourse to the 'facts' of the matter or the relevant evidence base; they are nevertheless involve decisions, which must be taken *in light* of the evidence (Hawkins and Parkhurst 2016). That is to say relevant research evidence is one component feeding into in a complex process of policy decision making. Evidence of the effects of policy problems will inform the prioritisation of issues, but cannot decide this in isolation from other values and contextual variables. Once a policy problem has been identified as a priority requiring a policy response, evidence will inform decisions about how to address an issue in the most (cost) effective way, but evidence alone cannot determine what course of action governments should take. Recognising both the political nature of decisions and the value of evidence to inform policy decisions (e.g. to ensure the efficacy and effectiveness and value for money of competing policy options) requires a more nuanced account of evidence which appreciates the role evidence can and cannot play in the identification and resolution of policy issues.

THE UK E-CIGARETTE POLICY DEBATE

These insights are of great relevance to the current UK e-cigarette debate in which policy actors often appear to be talking at cross purposes with each other. Whilst the basis of disagreements between policy actors appear to be routed in conflicts over evidence, the source of these disagreements lies in differing interpretations of the policy problem and the objectives of regulatory responses. Within the UK e-cigarette debate, actors have coalesced around what can be termed the 'harm-reduction' and 'population health' positons. By definition, the positions set out here and many actors will not fall squarely within either 'camp'. However, they are useful heuristics for discussing the different ways in which the issue is conceptualised and the nature of the controversy which has emerged.

The former consists of people actively involved in research and practise in the field of smoking cessations who prioritise the harm reduction potential of e-cigarettes for current smokers unwilling or unable to quit tobacco smoking. The logic of their position is that smokers may be able to transition away from smoking through e-cigarettes, reducing health harms experienced. The latter consist of people working in the broader areas of tobacco control and public health who prioritise concerns about the potentially negative population level effects of e-cigarettes and its potential to undermine current tobacco control policies. In addition, they question their efficacy as quit aids and assert the needs for a precautionary approach. Actors in both camps strongly assert the need for evidence based policy making, citing evidence which supports their position (cf. McNeill et al. 2015b; McKee and Capewell 2015a). The quality and policy implications of new studies which appear are highly contested.

The debates within the public health community are not conducted in isolation. There are other prominent participants in these regulatory debates whose concerns and interests overlap and contrast with those of the public health voices at different times in the debate. In particular, there is a prominent and apparently well organised e-cigarette user or 'vaper' movement which has engaged in policy debates to represent their preferences and interests as consumers. The transnational tobacco industry, which has aggressively entered the UK and global e-cigarette markets, has also sought to represent its interests in the debates. This is a source of great controversy given the well documented history of tobacco industry involvement both in the subversion of science and policy and in the co-opting of researchers and medical practitioners to confer legitimacy on its interventions (Brandt 2012). The presence of the tobacco industry in the debate, and the implications of this for tobacco control, is arguable the greatest source of controversy between different camps in the debate. The remainder of the chapter examines how these fundamentally different issue framings have led to significant disputes between policy actors in these camps and a range of topics relating to e-cigarette regulation: the potential health benefits of e-cigarettes; their classification as medical, tobacco or consumer devices; and the ways in which they should be marketed and smokers and non-smokers.

THE POTENTIAL HEALTH BENEFITS OF E-CIGARETTES

Policy debates on e-cigarettes turn on their potential health benefits. However, the way in which this is defined varies between camps. The debate on e-cigarettes has focused principally on the individual level health effects of e-cigarette use, and their harm reduction potential smoking for existing smokers (McNeill and Munafò 2013; Polosa et al. 2013; Cahn and Siegel 2011; Wagener et al. 2012; Riker et al. 2012). Whilst some argue, and cite evidence, that e-cigarettes are a less toxic alternative for smokers (Etter 2013; Wagener et al. 2012; McNeill and Munafò 2013; Polosa et al. 2013; Hajek et al. 2014), others have urged caution given the current uncertainty about their safety, usage patterns and their impact on existing tobacco control policies (Wagener et al. 2012; Taleb and Maziak 2013; Maziak 2014; Chapman 2014a). However, the health implications of long term vaping are uncertain, and it will require longitudinal studies of real world usage to establish its effects (Grana et al. 2014a).

The harm reduction potential of e-cigarettes turns on their ability to attract and retain smokers, who abandon cigarettes entirely, given that even radically reduced rates of smoking carry significant harms (Schane et al. 2010). To the extent that reduction in smoking through dual use with e-cigarettes this a precursor to quit attempts, this may also contribute to public health (Cheong et al. 2007). However, where dual use is continued and reduces quit attempts – through the false perception of reduced harm from decreased smoking or through the added convenience of being ability to 'vape' in smoke free environments – e-cigarette use may increase, not reduce, harm (Chapman 2014b). This in turn requires accurate assessments of usage patterns. Some limited evidence exists that e-cigarettes can aid smoking cessation. Whilst Brown et al. (2014) found them to be 60% more effective than nicotine replacement therapy (NRT) in quit attempts, Bullen et al. (2013) found e-cigarettes to be as effective as NRT. Further studies examine rates of e-cigarettes use (Evans and Hoffman 2014; Etter and Bullen 2014; Bullen et al. 2010, 2013), including amongst certain sub-groups including young people (Durmowicz 2014; Grana et al. 2014a; Maziak 2014) and those with mental health issues (Cummins et al. 2014).

Concerns have also arisen that e-cigarettes may act as a gateway to smoking, or entice ex-smokers to return to nicotine use (Zeller and Hatsukami 2009; Fairchild et al. 2014; Lee et al. 2014; Dutra and Glantz 2014; Grana et al. 2013; Maziak 2014). Whether the attractiveness of vaping (and, as will be discussed below, its marketing) to non-smokers is a cause for concern depends on the assessment of its harmfulness, as well as moral debates about the desirability of marketing a relatively unharmful, yet highly addictive, product such as nicotine to those who do not currently use it.

Those concerned with harm reduction have focussed on the relative toxicity of the e-cigarette vapour in comparison with tobacco smoke, both for consumers of these products and bystanders (Cahn and Siegel 2011; Goniewicz et al. 2013; Cheng 2014; Orr 2014; Callahan-Lyon 2014; Etter et al. 2011). Recent studies have also begun to address issues such as the availability of e-cigarettes (Rose et al. 2014), exposure to marketing (Huang et al. 2014; De Andrade and Hastings 2013a; Grana et al. 2014b) and the effects of that marketing on different groups (Emery et al. 2014; Pepper et al. 2014).

Others, meanwhile, have paid attention to the potential sociological effects of e-cigarettes through the renormalisation of smoking, and the circumvention of existing tobacco control measures, including advertising blackouts and clean air legislation (for exceptions see De Andrade and Hastings 2013a; Fairchild et al. 2014; Maziak 2014; Taleb and Maziak 2013; Zeller and Hatsukami 2009; Henningfield and Zaatari 2010). The similarity in appearance of many e-cigarettes and conventional cigarettes, as well as their packaging (Tobacco Tactics 2014b), may be used as a way for cigarette companies to circumvent cigarette advertising bans. Consequently, current debates appear to prioritise the issue of harm reduction for current smokers over measures designed to prevent the smoking uptake by future generations (Maziak 2014).

Classifying E-Cigarettes

Where e-cigarettes are legal products available for sale and consumption (e.g. in the UK), regulatory debates have focussed on whether e-cigarettes should be classified as medical devices, consumer goods or tobacco products. Public health advocates have argued in favour of their regulation as medical products, citing the precautionary principle and the absence of studies about their long term health effects. This approach, it is contended, is necessary in order to guarantee their safety and provide a framework for regulating marketing activities. Those favouring a harm reduction approach, meanwhile, have favoured a light-touch regulatory approach, seeing accessibility of products and the ease of transition to vaping as being key drivers of reduced smoking rates (Snowden 2013). Toxicity studies cited in the previous section are cited to support the framing of e-cigarettes as a safer alternative and the underline the importance of facilitating the transition of smokers to vaping. Proposals to regulate e-cigarettes as medical devices, it is claimed, both mischaracterise the product and preclude forms of marketing that would attract smokers to migrate to e-cigarettes (Gornall 2012; British American Tobacco 2013; Snowden 2013; Devlin 2012).

E-cigarettes are seen by their proponents as a 'market-led' solution to the smoking issue which must be differentiated form medicalised NRT, like gum or patches (Devlin 2012; Cahn and Siegel 2011; EC Forum Ltd. 2013). From this perspective, e-cigarettes are consumer products, aimed at those wishing to use nicotine recreationally without exposure to cigarette smoke (Snowden 2013). In part, this reflects a desire articulated by vociferous e-cigarette user groups in the debate to be seen not as sick people requiring treatment to recover from smoking, but as consumers choosing safer forms of nicotine consumption.

Marketing

In keeping with the differing visions of e-cigarettes as medical devices and consumer products, there are widely differing views on the forms of marketing which should be permitted for e-cigarettes. For those who see e-cigarettes as a potentially beneficial, market led phenomenon, attraction to these products through branding and promotion are an essential mechanism for reducing smoking by enticing smokers on to a safer alternative nicotine delivery mechanisms. On the other hand, concerns arise about the attractiveness of e-cigarette marketing for non-smokers and the wider public health effects of the promotion of vaping as a social practise.

E-cigarettes are now widely advertised and promoted online and in national media (Bauld et al. 2014; De Andrade and Hastings 2013b; Tobacco Tactics 2014b). Marketing materials often promote the harm reduction potential of their products for existing smokers (Richardson et al. 2014; De Andrade and Hastings 2013a). Citing the lower recorded level of toxins in e-cigarette vapour versus tobacco smoke (Goniewicz et al. 2013; Schripp et al. 2013), manufacturers claim they cause no long term harm to users, or to the air quality around them (Snowden 2013; Henningfield and Zaatari 2010; Hodgekiss 2013).

Critics have argued that e-cigarette manufacturers have made use of marketing techniques reminiscent of the tobacco industry, including celebrity endorsement and product placement in films and music videos

(Tobacco Tactics 2014b; De Andrade and Hastings 2013a). The proliferation of e-cigarette marketing via social media (Fallin et al. 2012; Grana et al. 2011), the introduction of flavoured products and claims that e-cigarettes are 'healthier' and environmentally friendly (Yamin et al. 2010; Fallin et al. 2012) have raised concerns they may be especially attractive to young consumers. Recent attempts to repackage and rebrand e-cigarettes, as "vapesticks" or brightly coloured "hookah pens," may be also appeal to youth (Richtel 2014). However, existing studies suggest levels of youth e-cigarette use remain low (McNeill et al. 2014).

Discussion and Conclusion

In the UK, significant divisions have opened up between policy actors highlighting the potentially positive and negative health effects of e-cigarette use and citing evidence which supports their positions. This issue has become particularly divisive within a public health community which had previously collaborated effectively on a consensual policy agenda.

A defining characteristic of this debate is the extent to which the lines of contestation are defined in terms of evidence and a strong normative commitment by actors on all sides to the goal of evidence based policy making. Policy actors on all sides point to evidence supporting their position and express frustration at the failure of others to follow the apparently self-evident policy prescriptions which follow from this. The apparent failure of their interlocutors to accept the facts presented and their policy consequences has led to accusations of bad faith and conflicts of interest to explain what is otherwise incomprehensible intransigence.

The analysis above compares the different positions articulated on specific aspects of the e-cigarette debate by policy actors and the evidence cited to support these. The two broad camps identified within the public health community are necessarily simplified interpretations of what is a more complex and nuanced array of different views but the division identified between the 'harm reduction' and 'public health' positions serves to demonstrate that different, at times mutually exclusive, positions on an issue such as e-cigarette policy can be support by relevant bodies of evidence. This is particularly the case with such novel products for which the research literature related to key policy issue is necessarily limited. It is erroneous, however, to assume that the current impasse can be overcome simply through the production of more evidence. In some instances, such as the long term health effects of e-cigarette use, consensus may emerge (as with the health effects of smoking) which deligitimises or marginalises certain policy positions. However, evidence alone will not be sufficient to resolve what are political and value driven controversies. Instead, what is needed to overcome the current divisions within public health, and with this a more coherent approach to developing effective and appropriate public policy, is a more explicit recognition of the political nature of the policy process and the possibility that multiple, competing framings of policy objects exist through a process of 'frame reflection' (Rein and Schön 1994). This may seem intuitive to social scientists, particularly those working in the realm of interpretative policy analysis. However, it is far more challenging for many public health actors whose training in the natural sciences perhaps does not equip them to recognise the existence of multiple competing narratives (and evidence bases) as a precursor to the process of frame reflection needed to overcome disputes. The natural science work on the assumptions of a single, universal 'truth', epistemologically accessible through the application of the correct methodology to the relevant data. The idea that there can be multiple interpretations of the same policy issue, multiple bodies of relevant evidence depending on those interpretations may run counter to their professional identities and their scholarly training. It may lead them to be oblivious to, or reject, the idea that there are multiple, competing 'truths' or problem definitions as a dangerous compromise or subversion of the scientific enterprise. However, this process of reflexivity about one's own position and assumptions which underpins processes of frame reflection, which will be essential in attempting to detoxify current debates and open up a space for engagement between actors at different ends of the debate.

REFERENCES

Abrams et al. 2014. *Statement from specialists in nicotine science and public health policy* [Online]. Available: http://www.webcitation.org/6ULpMDtvW. Accessed 8 Aug 2014.

Aktan et al. 2014. *129 public health and medical authorities from 31 countries write WHO DG Chan urging evidence-based approach to ecigs* [Online]. Available: http://www.webcitation.org/6ULpRXpPJ. Accessed 8 Aug 2014.

ASH. 2007. *UK tops the latest EU tobacco control league table* [Online]. Available: http://ash.org.uk/media-and-news/press-releases-media-and-news/uk-tops-the-latest-eu-tobacco-control-league-table/. Accessed 12 May 2017.

Bacchi, C. 2009. *Analysing policy: What's the problem representation to be*. Frenchs Forest: Pearson Education.
Bauld, L., K. Angus, and A.M. De. 2014. E-cigarette uptake and marketing: A report commissioned by Public Health England. *Public Health England*. Public Health England.
Bauld, L., A. Mcneill, P. Hajek, J. Britton, and M. Dockrell. 2016. E-cigarette use in public places: Striking the right balance. *Tobacco Control*, https://doi.org/10.1136/tobaccocontrol-2016-053357.
Brandt, A.M. 2012. Inventing conflicts of interest: A history of tobacco industry tactics. *American Journal of Public Health* 102: 63–71.
British American Tobacco. 2013. *A focus on harm Reuction: Why it matters* [Online]. Available: http://www.webcitation.org/6ULgu6oo3. Accessed 6 Nov 2013.
Brown, J., E. Beard, D. Kotz, S. Michie, and R. West. 2014. Real-world effectiveness of e-cigarettes when used to aid smoking cessation: A cross-sectional population study. *Addiction* 109: 1531.
Bullen, C., H. Mcrobbie, S. Thornley, M. Glover, R. Lin, and M. Laugesen. 2010. Effect of an electronic nicotine delivery device (e cigarette) on desire to smoke and withdrawal, user preferences and nicotine delivery: Randomised cross-over trial. *Tobacco Control* 19: 98–103.
Bullen, C., C. Howe, M. Laugesen, H. Mcrobbie, V. Parag, J. Williman, and N. Walker. 2013. Electronic cigarettes for smoking cessation: A randomised controlled trial. *The Lancet* 382: 1629–1637.
Cahn, Z., and M. Siegel. 2011. Electronic cigarettes as a harm reduction strategy for tobacco control: A step forward or a repeat of past mistakes. *Journal of Public Health Policy* 32: 16–31.
Cairney, P., and D. Studlar. 2014. Public health policy in the United Kingdom: After the war on tobacco, is a war on alcohol brewing? *World Medical & Health Policy* 6: 308–323.
Callahan-Lyon, P. 2014. Electronic cigarettes: Human health effects. *Tobacco Control* 23: ii36–ii40.
Chapman, S. 2013. Should electronic cigarettes be as freely available as tobacco cigarettes? No. *British Medical Journal* 346. Available: https://doi.org/10.1136/bmj.f3840.
———. 2014a. E-cigarettes: Does the new emperor of tobacco harm reduction have any clothes? *The European Journal of Public Health*. https://doi.org/10.1093/eurpub/cku054.
———. 2014b. E-cigarettes: The best and the worst case scenarios for public health—An essay by Simon Chapman. *British Medical Journal* 349: g5512.
Chapman, S., M. Daube, and W. Maziak. 2017. Should e-cigarette use be permitted in smoke-free public places? No. *Tobacco Control* 26: e3–e4.

Cheng, T. 2014. Chemical evaluation of electronic cigarettes. *Tobacco Control* 23: ii11–ii17.
Cheong, Y., H.-H. Yong, and R. Borland. 2007. Does how you quit affect success? A comparison between abrupt and gradual methods using data from the International Tobacco Control Policy Evaluation Study. *Nicotine & Tobacco Research* 9: 801–810.
Cummins, S.E., S.-H. Zhu, G.J. Tedeschi, A.C. Gamst, and M.G. Myers. 2014. Use of e-cigarettes by individuals with mental health conditions. *Tobacco Control* 23: iii48–iii53.
De Andrade, M., and G. Hastings. 2013a. *The marketing of e-cigarettes: A quick snapshot*. Cancer Research UK.
———. 2013b. Tobacco harm reduction and nicotine containing products: Research priorities and policy directions. *Social Marketing*. Cancer Research UK.
Devlin, K. 2012. *Response to BMA Briefing* [Online]. Available: http://www.ecita.org.uk/blog/index.php/response-to-bma-briefing/. Accessed 24 Jan 2014.
Dockrell, M., R. Morrison, L. Bauld, and A. McNeill. 2013. E-cigarettes: Prevalence and attitudes in Great Britain. *Nicotine and Tobacco Research* 15: 1737–1744.
Durmowicz, E.L. 2014. The impact of electronic cigarettes on the paediatric population. *Tobacco Control* 23: ii41–ii46.
Dutra, L.M., and S.A. Glantz. 2014. Electronic cigarettes and conventional cigarette use among US adolescents: A cross-sectional study. *JAMA Pediatrics* 168: 610.
EC Forum Ltd. 2013. *The E-cigarette summit: Science, regulation and public health*, November 12. London: The royal Society.
Emery, S.L., L. Vera, J. Huang, and G. Szczypka. 2014. Wanna know about vaping? Patterns of message exposure, seeking and sharing information about e-cigarettes across media platforms. *Tobacco Control* 23: iii17–iii25.
Etter, J.-F. 2013. Should electronic cigarettes be as freely available as tobacco? Yes. *British Medical Journal* 346: f3845.
Etter, J.-F., and C. Bullen. 2014. A longitudinal study of electronic cigarette users. *Addictive Behaviors* 39: 491–494.
Etter, J.-F., C. Bullen, A.D. Flouris, M. Laugesen, and T. Eissenberg. 2011. Electronic nicotine delivery systems: A research agenda. *Tobacco Control* 20: 243–248.
Evans, S.E., and A.C. Hoffman. 2014. Electronic cigarettes: Abuse liability, topography and subjective effects. *Tobacco Control* 23: ii23–ii29.
Fairchild, A.L., R. Bayer, and J. Colgrove. 2014. The renormalization of smoking? E-cigarettes and the tobacco "endgame". *New England Journal of Medicine* 370: 293.
Fallin, A., N.L. York, and E.J. Hahn. 2012. Tips for managing a social networking site. *Tobacco Control* 21: 507–508.

Gartner, C., and R.E. Malone. 2014. Duelling letters: Which one would you sign? *Tobacco Control* 23: 369–370.

Gneiting, U. 2015. From global agenda-setting to domestic implementation: Successes and challenges of the global health network on tobacco control. *Health Policy and Planning*. https://doi.org/10.1093/heapol/czv001.

Goniewicz, M.L., J. Knysak, M. Gawron, L. Kosmider, A. Sobczak, J. Kurek, A. Prokopowicz, M. Jablonska-Czapla, C. Rosik-Dulewska, and C. Havel. 2013. Levels of selected carcinogens and toxicants in vapour from electronic cigarettes. *Tobacco control*. https://doi.org/10.1136/tobaccocontrol-2012-050859.

Gornall, J. 2012. Electronic cigarettes: Medical device or consumer product? *British Medical Journal* 345: e6417.

Grana, R.A., S.A. Glantz, and P.M. Ling. 2011. Electronic nicotine delivery systems in the hands of Hollywood. *Tobacco Control* 20: 425–426.

Grana, R., N. Benowitz, and S.A. Glantz 2013. *Background paper on E-cigarettes* (electronic nicotine delivery systems). San Francisco: Center for Tobacco Control and Research and education.

Grana, R.A., P.M. Ling, N. Benowitz, and S. Glantz. 2014a. Electronic cigarettes. *Circulation* 129: e490–e492.

Grana, R.A., L. Popova, and P.M. Ling. 2014b. A longitudinal analysis of electronic cigarette use and smoking cessation. *JAMA Internal Medicine* 174: 812–813.

Hajek, P., J.F. Etter, N. Benowitz, T. Eissenberg, and H. Mcrobbie. 2014. Electronic cigarettes: Review of use, content, safety, effects on smokers and potential for harm and benefit. *Addiction* 109: 1801.

Hawkins, B., and J. Parkhurst. 2016. The 'good governance' of evidence in health policy. *Evidence & Policy* 12 (4): 575–592. https://doi.org/10.1332/174426 415x14430058455412.

Henningfield, J., and G. Zaatari. 2010. Electronic nicotine delivery systems: Emerging science foundation for policy. *Tobacco Control* 19: 89–90.

Hodgekiss, A. 2013. *Advert that claims electronic cigarette is 'completely harmless' banned as misleading* [Online]. London. Available: http://www.dailymail.co.uk/health/article-2262868/Advert-claims-electronic-cigarette-completely-harmless-banned-misleading.html. Accessed 23 Aug 2013.

Huang, J., R. Kornfield, G. Szczypka, and S.L. Emery. 2014. A cross-sectional examination of marketing of electronic cigarettes on Twitter. *Tobacco Control* 23: iii26–iii30.

Koon, A.D., B. Hawkins, and S.H. Mayhew. 2016. Framing and the health policy process: A scoping review. *Health Policy and Planning*. https://doi.org/10.1093/heapol/czv128.

Lancet, T. 2015. E-cigarettes: Public Health England's evidence-based confusion. *Lancet* 386: 829.

Lee, S., R.A. Grana, and S.A. Glantz. 2014. Electronic cigarette use among Korean adolescents: A cross-sectional study of market penetration, dual use, and relationship to quit attempts and former smoking. *Journal of Adolescent Health* 54: 684–690.

Majone, G. 1993. *Evidence argument and persuasion in the policy process.* New Haven: Yale University Press.

Manning, S. 2013. British American Tobacco enters electronic cigarette market in Britain with the 'Vype' [Online]. London. Available: http://www.independent.co.uk/news/uk/home-news/british-american-tobacco-enters-electronic-cigarette-market-in-britain-with-the-vype-8737286.html. Accessed 21 Aug 2013.

Maziak, W. 2014. Harm reduction at the crossroads: The case of E-cigarettes. *American Journal of Preventive Medicine* 47: 505–507.

McKee, M., and S. Capewell. 2015a. Electronic cigarettes: We need evidence, not opinions. *The Lancet* 386: 1239.

———. 2015b. Evidence about electronic cigarettes: A foundation built on rock or sand? *British Medical Journal* 351: h4863.

McNeill, A., and M.R. Munafò. 2013. Reducing harm from tobacco use. *Journal of Psychopharmacology* 27: 13–18.

McNeill, A., J.F. Etter, K. Farsalinos, P. Hajek, J. Houezec, and H. Mcrobbie. 2014. A critique of a WHO-commissioned report and associated article on electronic cigarettes. *Addiction* 109: 2128.

McNeill, A., L. Brose, R. Calder, S. Hitchman, P. Hajek, and H. Mcrobbie. 2015a. E-cigarettes: An evidence update. *Public Health England* 1–113. Available: https://assets.publishing.service.gov.uk/government/uploads/system/uploads/attachment_data/file/457102/Ecigarettes_an_evidence_update_A_report_commissioned_by_Public_Health_England_FINAL.pdf.

McNeill, A., L.S. Brose, R. Calder, S.C. Hitchman, P. Hajek, and H. Mcrobbie. 2015b. E-cigarettes: The need for clear communication on relative risks. *The Lancet* 386: 1237.

Orr, M.S. 2014. Electronic cigarettes in the USA: A summary of available toxicology data and suggestions for the future. *Tobacco Control* 23: ii18–ii22.

Parsons, W. 2002. From muddling through to muddling up-evidence based policy making and the modernisation of British government. *Public Policy and Administration* 17: 43–60.

Pepper, J.K., S.L. Emery, K.M. Ribisl, B.G. Southwell, and N.T. Brewer. 2014. Effects of advertisements on smokers' interest in trying e-cigarettes: The roles of product comparison and visual cues. *Tobacco Control* 23: iii31–iii36.

Polosa, R., B. Rodu, P. Caponnetto, M. Maglia, and C. Raciti. 2013. A fresh look at tobacco harm reduction: The case for the electronic cigarette. *Harm Reduction Journal* 10: 19.

Rein, M., and D. Schön. 1994. *Frame reflection. Towards the resolution of intractable policy controversies*. New York: Basic Books.
Richardson, A., O. Ganz, and D. Vallone. 2014. Tobacco on the web: Surveillance and characterisation of online tobacco and e-cigarette advertising. *Tobacco Control*. https://doi.org/10.1136/tobaccocontrol-2013-0501246.
Richtel, M. 2013. The E-cigarette Inductry, waiting to exhale [Online]. *New York Times*. Available: http://www.webcitation.org/6ULp7z7IL. Accessed 1 Nov 2013.
———. 2014. E-cigarettes, by other names, lure young and worry experts [Online]. *New York Times*. Available: http://www.nytimes.com/2014/03/05/business/e-cigarettes-under-aliases-elude-the-authorities.html?_r=0. Accessed 31 Mar 2014.
Riker, C.A., K. Lee, A. Darville, and E.J. Hahn. 2012. E-cigarettes: Promise or peril? *Nursing Clinics of North America* 47: 159–171.
Rose, S.W., D.C. Barker, H. D'angelo, T. Khan, J. Huang, F.J. Chaloupka, and K.M. Ribisl. 2014. The availability of electronic cigarettes in US retail outlets, 2012: Results of two national studies. *Tobacco Control* 23: iii10–iii16.
Schane, R.E., P.M. Ling, and S.A. Glantz. 2010. Health effects of light and intermittent smoking. *Circulation* 121: 1518–1522.
Schripp, T., D. Markewitz, E. Uhde, and T. Salthammer. 2013. Does e-cigarette consumption cause passive vaping? *Indoor Air* 23: 25–31.
Smith, K. 2013. *Beyond evidence based policy in public health: The interplay of ideas*. Basingstoke: Palgrave Macmillan.
Smithers, R. 2014. Whether they're called 'e-cigarettes' or 'vaporisers' the market is heating up [Online]. *The Guardian*. Available: http://www.theguardian.com/business/2014/jun/26/e-cigarettes-market-vaporisers. Accessed 8 Aug 2014.
Snowden, C. 2013. *Free market approaches to public health: The case of nicotine* [Online]. London: Institute of Economic Affairs. Available: http://www.iea.org.uk/sites/default/files/publications/files/Free%20Market%20Solutions%20in%20Health.pdf. Accessed 20 Aug 2013.
Stone, D.A. 1989. Causal stories and the formation of policy agendas. *Political Science Quarterly* 104: 281–300.
Taleb, Z.B., and W. Maziak. 2013. Harm reduction and e-cigarettes: Not evidence-based. *Regulation* 14: 1027.
Taylor, C. 1971. Interpretation and the sciences of man. *The Review of Metaphysics* 25: 3–51.
Thesing, G. 2014. Imperial Tobacco's Cooper adds Blu to take e-cigarette leap [Online]. *Bloomberg Business Week*. Available: http://www.businessweek.com/news/2014-07-15/imperial-tobacco-ceo-cooper-adds-blu-to-take-e-cigarette-leap. Accessed 8 Aug 2014.

Tobacco Tactics. 2014a. *E-cigarettes* [Online]. Tobacco Tactics. Available: http://www.tobaccotactics.org/index.php/E-cigarettes. Accessed 19 Sept 2014.

———. 2014b. *E-cigarettes: Marketing* [Online]. Available: http://www.tobaccotactics.org/index.php/E-cigarettes:_Marketing. Accessed 19 Sept 2014.

Van Hulst, M., and D. Yanow. 2016. From policy "frames" to "framing" theorizing a more dynamic, political approach. *The American Review of Public Administration* 46: 92–112.

Wagener, T.L., M. Siegel, and B. Borrelli. 2012. Electronic cigarettes: Achieving a balanced perspective. *Addiction* 107: 1545–1548.

Wipfli, H. 2015. *The global war on tobacco*. Baltimore: Johns Hopkins University Press.

World Health Organization. 2014. Electronic nicotine delivery systems: Report by WHO [Online]. Available: http://apps.who.int/gb/fctc/PDF/cop6/FCTC_COP6_10-en.pdf?ua=1. Accessed 17 Sept 2014.

Yamin, C.K., A. Bitton, and D.W. Bates. 2010. E-cigarettes: A rapidly growing internet phenomenon. *Annals of Internal Medicine* 153: 607–609.

Zeller, M., and D. Hatsukami. 2009. The strategic dialogue on tobacco harm reduction: A vision and blueprint for action in the US. *Tobacco Control* 18: 324–332.

Zhu, S.-H., J.Y. Sun, E. Bonnevie, S.E. Cummins, A. Gamst, L. Yin, and M. Lee. 2014. Four hundred and sixty brands of e-cigarettes and counting: Implications for product regulation. *Tobacco Control* 23: iii3–iii9.

Open Access This chapter is licensed under the terms of the Creative Commons Attribution 4.0 International License (http://creativecommons.org/licenses/by/4.0/), which permits use, sharing, adaptation, distribution and reproduction in any medium or format, as long as you give appropriate credit to the original author(s) and the source, provide a link to the Creative Commons license and indicate if changes were made.

The images or other third party material in this chapter are included in the chapter's Creative Commons license, unless indicated otherwise in a credit line to the material. If material is not included in the chapter's Creative Commons license and your intended use is not permitted by statutory regulation or exceeds the permitted use, you will need to obtain permission directly from the copyright holder.

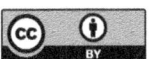

CHAPTER 8

Ministries of Health and the Stewardship of Health Evidence

Justin Parkhurst, Arturo Alvarez-Rosete, Stefanie Ettelt, Benjamin Hawkins, Marco Liverani, Elisa Vecchione, and Helen Walls

INTRODUCTION

This chapter brings together insights of parallel efforts to map out the structures and bodies providing evidence to inform health policy in the six GRIP-Health case study countries covered in this volume of work. More specifically, it reflects on the roles of Ministries of Health in each country, and the systems of evidence advice that provide policy relevant evidence to

---

J. Parkhurst (✉)
London School of Economics and Political Science, London, UK
e-mail: j.parkhurst@lse.ac.uk

A. Alvarez-Rosete • S. Ettelt • B. Hawkins • M. Liverani • E. Vecchione
• H. Walls
London School of Hygiene and Tropical Medicine, London, UK
e-mail: arturo.alvarez-rosete@lshtm.ac.uk; stefanie.ettelt@lshtm.ac.uk;
ben.hawkins@lshtm.ac.uk; marco.liverani@lshtm.ac.uk; e.vecchione@ucl.ac.uk;
helen.walls@lshtm.ac.uk

© The Author(s) 2018
J. Parkhurst et al. (eds.), *Evidence Use in Health Policy Making*,
International Series on Public Policy,
https://doi.org/10.1007/978-3-319-93467-9_8

these Ministries. This chapter describes how Ministries of Health have been mandated to act as stewards of populations' health according to the World Health Organization. We argue that this mandate extends to them having (at least partial) responsibility for ensuring relevant evidence and information informs health policy decisions. The chapter then discusses the need to consider evidence advisory systems serving Ministry needs, particularly considering whether or how such systems work to provide relevant and salient information in a timely manner to key decision points in the policy making process. Insights from our six cases are presented to illustrate the structural and practical differences which exist between evidence advisory systems and how, at certain times, key health decisions may in fact lie outside ministerial authority. These divergent experiences highlight a range of analytical challenges when considering the provision of evidence to inform health decisions from an institutional perspective. The following chapter continues the discussion with country case studies and comparative reflections on the use of evidence within government bodies outside Ministries of Health – particularly in the legislature and judiciary.

MINISTRIES AS STEWARDS OF HEALTH AND HEALTH EVIDENCE

A key debate in global health over the last two decades has concerned the role of the state in the health sector and in health systems governance (WHO 2000, p. 119; Saltman and Ferroussier-Davis 2000, p. 732; Reich 2002; Alvarez-Rosete 2008). This has grown in part from a renewed focus on the importance of health systems for improving population health, while simultaneously acknowledging the increasing diversity of decision-making forums and agencies involved in healthcare provision and implementation (Durán et al. 2011; Hafner and Shiffman 2012). (Dodgson et al. 2002) These changes have led to a shift in the vocabulary used by scholars. The term 'governance' began to replace 'government' within political science discourse since the 1990s, reflecting the decentred position of central government in public policy in many countries (Rhodes 1996, 1997; Kooiman 2000; Pierre 2000; Rosenau 1995; Stoker 1998).[1] These changes have occurred in parallel with the growing number of calls to ensure that health services, and wider health sector, planning is informed

---

[1] For overviews of this shift in terminology and focus, see: (Bell and Hindmoor 2009; Richards and Smith 2002; Piere and Peters 2000; Davies and Keating 2000; Kjaer 2011, 2004).

by the rigorous use of evidence, with a growing body of literature that has engaged with strategies to improve the uptake or use of evidence (c.f. van Kammen et al. 2006; LaRocca et al. 2012; Lavis et al. 2010). Yet in the changing health sector landscape, questions arise about whose role or responsibility it is to ensure health policy is informed by evidence.

Recent decades have also seen widespread debate about the capacity of the state to deliver policy outcomes and its right to intervene in the lives of the citizens it governs (Richards and Smith 2002; Bell and Hindmoor 2009). This shifting conceptualization of government as governance has also occurred in the arena of health (Dodgson et al. 2002; Kickbusch 2002; Lewis et al. 2006). Thus questions have been raised about the locus of political power in contemporary societies and whether the state enjoys the same degree of control and power over health systems and policy as in the past. (Bell and Hindmoor 2009; Bevir 2010; Rhodes 1997) In contemporary health systems, the number of old and new actors and institutions has multiplied, the boundaries between the public and private sectors have become more blurred, and central authorities' control over a much more complex policy process may now be challenged (Lewis et al. 2006; Alvarez-Rosete 2007; Saltman et al. 2011). The inherent complexity this implies means that such systems can only be governed through processes of steering, coordination and goal-setting for the range of different stakeholders involved and by developing a wide range of tools and strategies to this end.

The World Health Organization (WHO) introduced and championed the concept of *stewardship* of health systems as an essential government function in the year 2000 World Health Report (hereafter WHR 2000), which was devoted to the understanding, functioning and performance health systems. The report took a broad view of health systems as including: "all the organizations, institutions and resources that are devoted to producing health actions. [Continuing:] A health action is defined as any effort, whether in personal health care, public health services or through intersectoral initiatives, whose primary purpose is to improve health (p. xi)".

The WHR 2000 is widely held up by the health community as a key document championing and reinvigorating the focus on health systems, with ministries of health being seen as health system stewards. Many subsequent WHO reports and policies have aimed at strengthening systems as well as the institutional mechanisms for governing them (WHO 2003, 2007, 2008). Similarly, WHO regional offices have had the intertwined topics of health systems development and state governance roles at the heart of their discussions (WHOROE 2008; Kickbusch and Gleicher 2012) – also see (McQueen et al. 2012).

The terms *governance* and *stewardship* have often been used as synonyms by those working in the health field, yet stewardship implies a particular mandate, and ultimate responsibility, for population health that is reflected when the WHO states:

> The ultimate responsibility for the overall performance of a country's health system lies with government, which in turn should involve all sectors of society in its stewardship [...] The health of the people is always a national priority: government responsibility for it is continuous and permanent. Ministries of health must therefore take on a large part of the stewardship of health systems. (WHO 2000, p. xiv)

According to the WHR 2000, such responsibility is exercised over three distinct dimensions of stewardship (p. 122):

- Formulating health policy – defining the vision and direction;
- Exerting influence – approaches to regulation;
- Collecting and using intelligence.

Whilst the first two components indicate a responsibility to oversee health policy and the conduct of health actors, the third dimension – 'collecting and using intelligence' – captures many of the common ideas about the use of policy relevant information to inform health decisions.

INSTITUTIONAL SYSTEMS OF EVIDENCE ADVISE FOR HEALTH POLICY

Ministries of Health may thus be seen as having a mandate over decisions affecting the health of the people, as well as over the use of evidence and information to guide those decisions. However, effective utilisation of evidence requires a conduit through which it can reach relevant decision-makers at times when such information can be useful. Thus applying wider 'governance' concepts to the question of evidence use, it becomes clear that Ministries will not necessarily take it upon themselves to gather and analyse all policy relevant evidence (although some of them may try to). Rather, they can serve as the *stewards of health evidence* by overseeing and maintaining the institutional arrangements in place which serve to provide policy-relevant evidence.

Ministries can rely on a more or less formalised network of bodies and groups to serve as the providers of policy-relevant evidence (Nutley et al. 2007; Parkhurst 2017) – networks we refer to as 'evidence advisory systems', which can be seen to reflect a specific form of the broader concept of 'policy advisory systems' within the public policy literature. According to Hustedt and Veit (2017), "The concept of policy advisory systems focuses on the country-specific organization and institutionalization of policy advice. It refers to an interlocking set of actors with a unique configuration in each sector and jurisdiction, who provide information, knowledge, and recommendations for actions to policy-makers" (p. 42).

One of the first authors to explicitly discuss policy advisory bodies from an institutional perspective was John Halligan (1995) who explored the location of the body providing advice (within the public service, internal to the government, or external) and reflected on the level of government control each might entail. Halligan notes that there is no consensus as to the 'best' structure for policy advice, but highlights some of the different potential issues that might be raised by differing systems, including the level of independence of the advisory bodies or the level of public consultation involved. He proposes three principles that might be seen as central to a good advisory system, however: the provision of multiple sources of advice; the flexibility to be able to choose a mix of advisors and processes appropriate to a particular issue; and an explicit concern with the effectiveness of advice.

More recently, scholars have questioned whether Halligan's focus on location of advice is necessarily the best factor to consider when judging policy advisory systems. Craft and Howlett (2012), for instance, argue that this focus may ignore a number of other key concerns to those studying advisory systems, including the content of the policy advice itself, which can have important implications for the kinds of decisions advice that is being provided. Other scholars have started to investigate policy advisory systems in greater depth, but according to Hustedt and Veit (2017), much of this work has focussed on western democracies, looking at questions such as the externalisation of advice or politicisation of advice, with a large number of other policy-relevant questions remaining unaddressed. In the health sector, Koon and colleagues (Koon et al. 2013) have more specifically discussed the importance of 'embeddedness' of health policy and systems research to inform health policy decisions; with embeddedness reflecting the centrality and networked links these forms of research have in various government systems.

However, the explicit normative goal of Ministries of Health to serve in a stewardship role to improve population health provides a useful lens by which to analyse evidence advisory systems. Indeed, while high level legislatures and political bodies may see their ultimate goals continually being debated or changed as political priorities shift, Ministries of Health typically have a fairly commonly agreed set of goals that can be used to reflect on how evidence advisory systems in place work to serve those needs or achieve health sector goals.

Indeed, stakeholders calling for increased or improved uses of evidence in health policy typically make such calls on the basis of a set of (stated or unstated) assumptions. First, the goals of health policy to improve population health – primarily though reducing morbidity and mortality, extending life expectancy, or decreasing health inequalities – are taken as given by many public health advocates. Furthermore, the particular emphasis on scientific evidence is based on an underlying assumption that more rigorous and systematic uses of evidence are likely to lead to greater effectiveness and efficiency than piecemeal or scientifically flawed uses of evidence (Chalmers 2003; Chalmers et al. 2002; Parkhurst 2017). Yet efficiency gains of this nature further require that policy-relevant evidence is produced and reaches the appropriate decision making body in a timely manner in order to be usable. These criteria provide us with a lens through which to evaluate the structures, functions and effectiveness of evidence advisory bodies serving Ministries of Health.

HEALTH DECISIONS AND NEEDS

The public policy literature recognises that the term 'policy' can refer to a range of concepts, from projects and programmes, to sector-specific plans, to broad statements of intent (Hogwood and Gunn 1984). Policy is also rarely the responsibility of a single body; rather, policy decisions affecting health take place at difference levels of governance (i.e. sub-national, national and supra-national) across a range of state and non-state decision making forums. As such, the most relevant forms of evidence will vary across policy issues and decision types of policy-making location.

However, there are some types of decisions common to many countries' health sectors for which research evidence is often held as critical, and over which Ministries of Health typically are seen to have authority. This allows a basic typology of decision types to provide a starting point to explore how evidence advisory systems work to provide policy-relevant evidence. For example:

- Public health and health promotion: Decisions of this kind are usually done at a high level as they affect large segments of the population. A broad range of evidence will thus be relevant to such decisions, including epidemiological, economic, social attitude, and other data which speak to relevant policy concerns.
- Health sector planning and priority setting: These decisions are concerned with setting national goals and priority setting across the sector. They can also involve allocation of resources between local health concerns. Relevant evidence forms can thus include population health data, resource health technology appraisals/assessments (HTA), or health services research.
- Health systems and services management: In addition to new policy decisions and priority setting, Ministries of Health also typically make ongoing decisions related to the management and functioning of the health system. Relevant evidence can include routine data collected from facilities or surveys, operations research, implementation research, or other programmatic evidence.
- Programmatic decision making: What many authors refer to as health policy decisions fall within the remit of specialised agencies, such as programmes dedicated to individual conditions (cancer, HIV/AIDS, malaria, etc.). In particular these decisions can involve the choice of interventions to pursue, often with a fixed budget to allocate. Decisions of this nature can require evidence both about efficacy or cost effectiveness of available options, but equally can be informed by locally generated data (e.g. routine data from surveillance or facility information).

Even within these broad categories, decision making for health can take place at different levels within government hierarchies, with authority for decisions, and entry points for evidence, resting in national level bodies and sub-national bodies. In different country settings the various decision types listed above might be addressed at any level or may cut across more than one. Moreover, they may be shaped by supra-national policy regimes (such as those of the European Union). Movements towards de-centralisation might also lead to the shifting of decision-making from national levels to lower levels. Such realities, however, allow consideration of whether systems of evidentiary advice are well aligned with the decision authority structures in a given setting. There can also be important considerations on the ways that national evidence systems link to influential non-state decision makers (e.g. development partners in low and middle income settings, or corporatist bodies with authority in health decision making fora).

COUNTRY CASE STUDIES

In each case study country, members of the GRIP-Health research programme attempted to map out the key health policy decision making bodies, and the sources of evidence in the country that inform health decisions. These mappings allowed reflection on how the evidence advisory system in each country might work, or face challenges, in aligning sources of policy relevant evidence with the policy needs in each setting. The subsections below summarise some of the key findings from each case. This is then followed by a discussion of cross cutting issues and themes seen from multiple settings.

Ghana

In Ghana, the Ministry of Health (MoH) provides overall policy direction for all stakeholders and players in the health sector, and approves health decisions related to specific health system issues, including health system strengthening and, at times, programme or disease specific interventions. The Ghana Health Service (GHS) is an autonomous Executive Agency of the MoH which has been delegated the responsibility to manage and operate all public health facilities (except for three teaching hospitals); while the National Health Insurance Authority (NHIA) is also the primary body which decides on the package of services available to many citizens.

Ghana has established some formal internal bodies to provide evidence to these agencies. Within the GHS, the Policy, Planning, Monitoring and Evaluation division and the Research & Development division are both tasked with evidence generation. The GHS also hosts the Centre for Health Information Management which includes the District Health Information Management System, through which routine health data (administrative, demographic and clinical) is provided from local facilities to districts and upwards to central health management levels. In the MoH there is also a Research, Statistics and Information Management Directorate and a MoH-based Policy, Planning, Monitoring and Evaluation division as well which are responsible for generating evidence and advising the MoH. The GHS also directs three regional research centres that conduct health services and systems research within their designated areas to guide national decision making.

In these ways, Ghana appears to have a well-aligned bureaucracy providing relevant research and evidence to key decision making bodies. However we did identify some challenges and further needs as well. First, as a lower-middle income country, there were some expected capacity limitations in terms of volume of research and population of experts to provide relevant evidence. Furthermore, while the NHIA is tasked with choosing the services covered by the National Health Insurance Scheme, the GHS decides the NHIS charges at each facility. Interviews and participatory observations at the annual business meeting with international partners in November 2015, identified a latent rivalry between the two government agencies due to conflicting interests in generating and using evidence to inform decisions as purchaser (NHIA) and provider (GHS) of health services.

At the time of research, there was not any formalised or fully agreed system of Health Technology Appraisal (HTA) in place to guide decisions on health services provided across the health sector, although there was some movement towards using HTA to inform individual decisions. Funding for many health programmes is also reliant on international donors (so called 'development partners'), which was said to lead to vertical programming independent of any evidence of local priorities or need. International donors were also said to use their own systems and bodies of evidence at times.

Reliance on development partners, who can retain decision making authority in some ways, can thus pose challenges to rationalising evidence use and ensuring local stewardship of evidence advisory systems. On the one hand, donors obviously provide finance for health services, and will no doubt at times be undertaking evaluations of programmes that can generate policy relevant evidence. Yet, such systems are external to national structures, and thus risk establishing parallel systems of evidence advisory outside those under the control of, and at the service of, national authorities.

Finally, it was identified that the Ghanaian Parliament had a remit to make decisions around health financing nationally and other health related legislation through the Parliament select committee on health. However, local interviewees noted limited influence of this committee due to financial constraints prohibiting its ability to gather information or undertake inquiries as needed. Also, the involvement of local MPs into the two annual business meetings with development partners is limited, with consequent inability to obtain relevant information on future health interventions and leverage their positions at the moment of approving the government budget.

Colombia

Colombia is the second middle income case study country, included yet its differences with Ghana illustrate just how context-specific health policy-making can be. Since the inception of the Colombian health system in 1993, highly politicised disagreements have been sustained on issues such as the financing of the system (insurance versus taxation based); the involvement of the private sector; and whether limits can or should be placed on the right to health care. Policy debates almost exclusively focus on macro/systemic health sector reforms, to the exclusion of many other health policy issues.

As an insurance based health system, the Ministry of Health and Social Protection (*Ministerio de Salud y Protección Social, MSPS*) primarily steers health care by setting the mandatory basic service package (the Plan Obligatorio de Salud [POS]) and regulating the system; although it does not have a direct managerial input on health care facilities. However, roles and authority over these functions have also changed or been assigned (or reassigned) between the Ministry and other bodies in recent years. For instance from 2007 a Regulatory Commission for Health was set up to update the package of health services provided in Colombia, but in 2012 it was abolished and the Ministry re-assumed this role (Castro 2014).

The health policy decision making process in Colombia also involves a range of different institutions across the branches of government as well as non-state actors (e.g. civil society organisations, health insurers, service providers, academia and professional organisations). The governance of the health system is thus extremely fragmented, reflecting the complexity of the health system itself (Bernal et al. 2012; Yamin and Parra-Vera 2010). Furthermore, the judiciary plays a particularly important role in health policymaking in Colombia (as discussed in more depth in Chap. 5) as it often serves as the means by which the public challenges insurers on what should be included in the package of services.

The Ministry does have a series of organizations ascribed to it with responsibilities for evidence provision through their mandate to advise on decisions in health, including: the Instituto Nacional de Salud (INS) (the National Health Institute); the Instituto de Evaluación de Tecnologíca en

Salud (IETS) (Institute of Health Technology Assessment); and the Instituto Nacional de Vigilancia de Medicinas y Alimentos (INVIMA) (National Institute for the Vigilance of Medicines and Food). Yet there is no unique central hub of evidence generation in the Ministry; instead, each unit and directorate within the Ministry appears to be responsible for its own areas of expertise; and these national advisory bodies may thus have limited influence given the fragmented governance of decision making, providing advice to some decision points but not necessarily others.

Overall, some of the biggest challenges to the use of evidence for health policy thus includes the fragmentation of decision making, the politicisation over fundamental elements of health care provision (diverting time and attention away from more specific health service and systems planning) and the lack of central authority vested in the Ministry of Health and Social Protection. In combination, these factors limit how much evidence advisory bodies can influence health policy decisions in 'rational-technical' ways often expected by public health advocates.

Cambodia

Cambodia was selected as one of our low income setting cases at the time of research, although today it is classified as 'lower-middle income' in World Bank rankings. Despite recent economic growth, it still has limited state provision of health services. Estimates vary, but survey data suggest two-thirds of health spending is financed by consumer out-of-pocket payments ([Cambodia] National Institute of Statistics Directorate for Health 2015), with national demographic and health surveys suggesting only one-fifth of treatments carried out by the public sector.

The MoH has the mandate to monitor the country's health status, advise central government on health policies and legislation, formulate strategies and develop programmes to address the country's health problems, and implement, monitor and evaluate all health programmes and activities in the country in collaboration with other sectors and agencies. There are also numerous national programmes, centres and institutions important to the Cambodian health system, many of which are issue specific in their remit. These include the National Maternal and Child Health Centre (NMCH), the National Centre for HIV/AIDS, Dermatology and STD (NCHADS) and the National Institute of Public Health (NIPH). These technical health departments and national centres sit within the MoH structure, and can initiate specific health policies or guidelines

(Jones and Camboida Economic Associate Centre for Policy Studies 2013). The Ministry of Economics and Finance (MEF) was noted to be one of the most important other decision making bodies in Cambodia affecting health, however, as it is responsible for financing the health system, and particularly important for health policy decisions with budgetary implications in the country. International development partners (donors) are also highly influential in the Cambodian health sector as over half of the public budget is funded by aid (approximately 52% of the health budget, as estimated in 2011 (World Bank 2011)). Local respondents further noted that research topics are heavily driven by external funders, rather than assessments of health policy priorities by local bodies.

Whilst there appears to be a demand for evidence and research in health policy-making in Cambodia, including language used within Ministry documents of a need for 'evidence based' approaches, this demand does not appear to be deeply embedded in MoH systems and structures. A considerable amount of research is produced in the sector in the form of reviews and assessments for specific projects or programmes. This work is often conducted by commissioned consultancies, and has been described elsewhere by Jones (2013) to be of variable quality. Jones further notes concern over the supply of policy-relevant data in the country (Jones and Camboida Economic Associate Centre for Policy Studies 2013). Some information sources (or documents collecting data) are institutionalised, however. For example, the annual operational plan (AOP) process and the health management information system (HMIS); although private consultations and treatments (accounting for about 70% of care) are not captured in the HMIS. Indeed, the Ministry itself has highlighted the need to improve the reliability and policy relevance of the system (Cambodia Ministry of Health 2008). Furthermore it was reported that the Ministry had no way to monitor or gather data from most private providers of health services, despite this capturing a majority of treatment in the country. The domestic research community is also relatively weak in regard to health, particularly due to limited funding and the low strategic importance accorded to research by political actors (Jones and Camboida Economic Associate Centre for Policy Studies 2013).

In terms of technical bodies, the National Institute for Public Health (NIPH) is one of the most notable within the Cambodian system. It is a semi-autonomous institute under the MoH tasked to undertake research, knowledge translation, and training – although it has reportedly largely focused on training, as no budget has been provided for research activities.

Given these resource constraints, including limited staffing capacity, the NIPH is not currently considered a strong player in the domestic research community. However, it does appear to have a clear mandate and institutional position to serve an evidence advisory role.

In terms of donor-funded evidence use, research projects are often focussed on programme evaluation. They have often been critiqued for lacking coordination, resulting in duplications of efforts and inefficient use of resources, and lacking integration in terms of data collection and analysis (Jones and Camboida Economic Associate Centre for Policy Studies 2013). There are some efforts to coordinate data and evidence to inform national level strategic planning, however. In particular, the drafting of the Health Strategic Plan, the mid-term review process of the Plan, as well as annual performance reviews are supported by consultation mechanisms in which data are presented and discussed. Most notable is the Technical Working Group for Health, chaired by the Minster of Health, which brings together government and development partners to present and discuss evidence to inform this high level of sector planning and review.

The evidence advisory system for health policy-making in Cambodia thus appears to suffer from limited capacity and a vertical programme orientation – often driven by sources of funds from outside actors (e.g. donors). There is a lack of strategy in the handling of the evidence and knowledge base for the health sector, and management and decision-making based on research evidence and analysis is limited in both health policy-making and service delivery. However, policy makers are aware of the need to develop a research agenda for the sector (expressed in interviews and seen in MoH documents identifying needed improvements), and some MoH working groups have increasingly been giving attention to this issue. There are also existing institutional bodies that could serve more central or relevant roles in evidence generation or synthesis in the future, with greater capacity and integration into planning processes.

Ethiopia

Ethiopia served as our second low income case. The country is officially a federation, and the constitution establishes dual jurisdiction over public health between the Federal and the Regional governments. However, the Federal Ministry of Health has control over the national health policy, formulating the national strategic plan for the health sector. Since 1991, Ethiopia has made improvements to health care delivery and set the basic foundations of a health system, improvements that are recognized by some as a success story of health system reform (Downie 2016). In this process, the role of health research has been seen to be critical; consequently, Ethiopia has at times made explicit commitments to improving the use of evidence in health (c.f. Ethiopian Academy of Science 2013).

Given the limited resources in country, there have been expected ongoing challenges in terms of low research-related technical and human capacity and an absence of strong research priority-setting mechanisms. Yet these limitations seem not to have undermined the capacity of the Federal Ministry of Health (FMoH) to make decisions in health and enforce commitments with development partners (Downie 2016). Instead, the government of Ethiopia appears to have maintained a strong central controlling function over the decisions which have been made. Health policymaking in Ethiopia appears heavily focussed on centralised planning, and particularly draws on routine data sources to inform decisions. Data gathering and analysis are concentrated in two main national agencies, the Central Statistical Agency and the recently reorganised Ethiopian Public Health Institute. Data on health facilities are collected at the community level, then reported to the district (*woreda*), regional and national levels. The FMoH then uses data to produce indicators that are passed back to lower levels to elaborate local health plans (Ethiopia Federal Ministry of Health 2014).

The bureaucratic structures in Ethiopia thus appear to be well aligned for this collection and review of local data for planning. The Policy and Planning Directorate within the FMoH hosts the Health Management Information System (HMIS), for instance, which is a key component of the system. According to national documents, the HMIS is also used to identify funding gaps and priorities in order to inform the need for donor assistance (Ethiopia Federal Ministry of Health 2014).

Generation and review of other forms of evidence to inform planning decisions, however, do show limitations. For example, the Ethiopia Public Health Institute serves as a semi-autonomous institution under the FMOH and is the technical arm of the FMOH. Its main tasks are to undertake research on priority health and nutrition problems and on public health emergencies management. Yet the capacity of this body was said to be limited, leading to fairly piecemeal production of policy relevant evidence. For example, a representative from the Technology Transfer and Research Translation Directorate of EHPI noted that there were very few staff to undertake activities, and only a few policy briefs had been produced to inform decision making at that time.

It is therefore generally indicated that evidence production and use in Ethiopia are still limited, mainly due to insufficient human capacity in generating evidence and in the relatively young establishment of the culture of evidence-informed policy-making (African Health Observatory 2014). Consolidating and publishing existing evidence for policy-making and decision-making has thus been described as limited and unsystematic (Gaym 2008). Yet this stands in contrast to the seemingly well established and centrally controlled system of planning around routine data sources in the country.

England

England represents the first of our high income case study settings. The country is well known for its tax funded and state provided National Health Service (NHS). Elements of evidence use within the English system are also often held up as exemplars of evidence informed policy. In particular, the National Institute for Health and Care Excellence (NICE) – a non-departmental public body that provides clinical guidelines and health technology appraisals for the NHS – has been held up as a role model both domestically and internationally. Within England, it has served as the inspiration for a set of 'what works' centres that aim to emulate the health approach to synthesising evidence of interventions to inform policymaking (UK Government 2013). Globally it has been a template for health technology assessment bodies in other countries (Including Colombia as noted above, and described by Castro (2014) elsewhere).

The Department (Ministry) of Health has overall responsibility for the NHS, public health and social care, within a legislative framework set by Parliament. The Department is supported by 26 agencies and public bodies. Of these, 15 are referred to as 'arm's-length bodies', with different degrees of independence from government. The remaining bodies are advisory non-departmental public bodies, whose role is to assist the Department in "evaluating, investigating and supporting policy" and providing independent scientific expertise (Boyle 2011). The Department is also supported by two executive agencies: the Medicines and Healthcare products Regulatory Agency (MHRA), responsible for regulating medicines, medical devices and blood components for transfusion, and Public Health England (PHE), developing public health and health promotion policy. Finally, NICE is a non-departmental body that provides national guidance and advice for health, public health and social care practitioners, as well as quality standards for the provision and the commissioning of these services. This includes the appraisal of new medical technologies using principles of cost-effectiveness (NICE 2017). NICE therefore plays a key role in defining the package of services available to patients in the NHS.

In general, scientific evidence plays a pivotal role in the governance of the NHS. There is a substantial volume of health systems, health services and health policy research produced in the UK (in addition to clinical research and basic sciences) which has led some authors to describe a culture of evidence use in which the NHS aims to become, a "consistent, evidence-based whole (Shergold and Grant 2008, p. 7)" with substantial 'absorptive capacity' for publicly and privately-funded health research (Hanney et al. 2010).

The evidence advisory system, however, combines multiple elements. In Parliament, select committees play a key role in holding the government to account for its decisions, policies, and reforms; and they mostly do so in relation to health policy through an assessment of the available evidence base. The Department of Health, however, has a history of commissioning research on behalf of the NHS, PHE and others, and of collaborating with the various government research bodies that fund health related research. The National Institute of Health Research (NIHR) was created in 2006, and coordinates research efforts to inform the health system. Finally, England is a leading market for think tanks, including in the health sector. However it has been argued that little is known about how such think tanks prioritize topics, fund their research (and the methodologies employed), or influence health policy-making; with calls for greater research into their roles and biases in health policy-making (Shaw et al. 2014). Despite this, overall the English system has widely been seen as a strong example of a coordinated evidence advisory system that attempts to institutionalise evidence use in health policy and health system governance.

Germany

Germany represents our final case study country and second high income setting, but one that looks very different from England in its health system structure and broader governance approach. One of the most relevant features, perhaps, is how much health decision making takes place outside the remit of the Ministry of Health. Germany is a federal parliamentary republic comprised of 16 states (*Länder*). The Basic Law (*Grundgesetz*) provides for the separation of powers between the *Bund* (federal state) and the *Länder* and sets out their respective rights and responsibilities. The Basic Law also sets out the general principles that shape health system governance, including a commitment to 'corporatism' – which broadly involves governance through power sharing with major interest groups. Responsibilities for health system governance are thus shared by federal, states and municipalities, as well as the corporatist self-administration.

Parliamentary decision-making is prepared by, and largely happens in, committees. For health policy, two standing committees are most relevant: the Health Committee (*Gesundheitsausschuss*) and the Conciliation Committee (*Vermittlungsausschuss*). Health care legislation, including major health care reform, is usually initiated by the federal minister of health. The main responsibility of the Federal Ministry of Health is to maintain, secure and advance an effective statutory health system ([Germany] Federal Ministry of Health 2015). The Federal Ministry of Health has several ways of steering health and health care policy: developing legislation, decrees and administrative directives; supervising the provision of tasks that have been delegated to the self-administration; and co-ordinating stakeholders in health system governance in other ways, for example, through organising initiatives, establishing committees or promoting other forms of collaborative work.

However, in line with the Basic Law, a large number of decision-making and regulatory tasks have been delegated to the organisations of the self-administration. At federal level, key corporatist actors are the top organisations of sickness funds (*Spitzenverband der deutschen Krankenkassen*), representing public payers, the German Hospital Association (*Deutsche Krankenhausgesellschaft*) and the federal association of office-based doctors and dentists who deliver services funded by social health insurance (*Kassenärztliche Bundesvereinigung*). Within this self-administration, the Federal Joint Committee (GBA) is the highest decision-making body at federal level, composed of these federal associations.

The Federal Ministry of Health is advised by a number of permanent or temporary expert committees. Permanent committees are the Advisory Council on the Assessment of Developments in the Health Care System and the Joint Scientific Council of the Agencies and Institutes, subordinate to the Ministry. Both committees largely consist of scientific experts. The Federal Ministry of Health also has administrative oversight of a number of federal agencies and research institutes, but research commissioned directly by the Ministry is limited.

In contrast, the use of scientific evidence is central for the GBA. Scientific evidence plays a key role in many, but not all, decisions of the GBA and practices of using evidence are embedded in the rules of procedures set out in the GBA's by-laws. Two research institutes support the work of the GBA: The Institute for Quality and Efficiency in Health Care (IQWiG), established in 2004, and the Institute for Quality Assurance and Transparency in Health Care (IQTIG), which became operational in 2016. IQWiG, for instance, is mandated to provide health technology assessments and reviews of scientific evidence in relation to the efficacy of pharmaceuticals, diagnostics and medical treatment, evidence-based clinical guidelines and patient information.

However, given its broad remit and the diversity of its regulatory tasks, scientific evidence will be used in different ways for different types of decisions by the GBA. This will depend on the nature of the issue, the types, quality and quantity of studies available, the availability of (international) standards of evidence use (e.g. clinical guidelines, health technology assessment), and the degree to which the issue affects stakeholder interests. As a result, decisions concerning the funding of health technologies, such as pharmaceuticals, diagnostics and medical treatments are typically robustly supported by evidence, while decisions concerning distributional issues such as the geographical coverage of physicians in the ambulatory sector (i.e. capacity planning) show fewer traces of scientific analysis and are more likely to be the product of negotiation between the interest groups represented on the committee. However, in contrast to NICE in England, decisions concerning the package of service do not utilise evidence of cost-effectiveness as a criterion for funding decisions.

Many other organisations of the self-administration, especially at the federal level (e.g. the Sickness Funds, or Federal Association of Physicians), have developed their own research capacity and/or are supported by their own research institutes. These take a variety of organisational and legal forms, and some may be more independent from the organisation commissioning the research than others.

Overall, Germany has deeply rooted systems of democratic accountability, but the decentralised nature of the state limits the stewardship role of the federal government, including the Federal Ministry of Health (BMG), to influence health policy and health service governance. As health system governance is spread across a number of state and non-state actors, there is no single mechanism of decision-making and therefore no single entry point for scientific research. Consequently, there are multiple conduits for scientific evidence to enter the policy process, be it in parliament, federal government, the self-administration and its member organisations, and the legal system; with a large number of research institutes, scientific advisory bodies, expert committees and other mechanisms providing scientific advice. However, there are few formal rules that require decision-making to be informed by scientific evidence, with explicit procedures for evidence use in decisions taken by the GBA on inclusions to or exclusions from the statutory benefits package being an exception rather than a norm.

Discussion: Issues and Challenges

The six countries included in the GRIP-Health programme of work represent a wide range of health policy contexts – ranging from low to high income, covering four continents, and having widely divergent historical and political experiences and socioeconomic profiles. However, in all cases there are core health systems decisions that need to be made, and structures in support of providing evidence to inform such decisions. In all cases (with the possible exception of Germany), Ministries of health were found to be central to these forms of decisions; although we also identified situations where decision authority lies outside the Ministry.

From an institutional perspective, we have particularly focussed on the evidence advisory systems that inform key health policy decisions in each country setting. Each country is of course unique in the historical development of its health systems and associated bureaucracy. As such, we would not expect evidence advisory systems to necessarily look the same across these contexts. Rather, they will have been established, by default or design, within pre-existing administrative structures – products of their specific history which shapes the potential directions and features of any systems being developed. The ultimate goals of improving health and health decision making, however, can be where we look for similarities and comparisons. In particular, it can be assumed that, for evidence advisory systems to function effectively, they must be able to provide robust and high quality syntheses of different forms of evidence, relevant to the specific policy issue at hand, to the appropriate decision makers or bodies responsible for policy decisions which can use them in a timely manner to inform relevant health decisions. We can thus reflect, in a comparative perspective across case study countries, on the alignment of these systems with the decision making needs of the health sector – and of Ministries of

Health in particular – given these ministries mandate as stewards of population health, and a recognised need for these bodies to use information to inform decisions.

Decisions on Packages of Services

One theme we can see arising in multiple countries is the central concern across case study countries with the package of health care services to provide to the public – either through state provided health facilities, or within packages of services included in state-regulated insurance programmes. Comparing our case studies illustrates some particular issues with the institutional arrangements in place to supply evidence to inform these decisions. It was in our middle income cases (Colombia and Ghana) where the challenges in the systems to inform such decisions were most visible. Indeed, in the lower income settings studied (Ethiopia and Cambodia), local stakeholders did not raise these decisions as primary concerns in interviews – potentially due to the inability to provide comprehensive packages of care in the first place. When needs are well beyond resources available, and funds for services are highly dependent on both donors and individuals' out of pocket expenditures, there may be little perceived need to have an evidence base on which to judge inclusion or exclusion of a formal package of services. Alternatively, in our high income settings (England and Germany), there were already well established formal systems informing these decisions, albeit very different in structure. There are also notable differences in the type of evidence included in such decisions between both countries, with NICE in England basing its recommendations on cost effectiveness, a criterion which is absent from the German regulatory approach.

In our middle income settings, decisions about the package of health services were indeed being made, but without a fully established structure to provide evidence to inform such decisions. In Ghana, the National Health Insurance Agency (NHIA) has had to decide what to include in its service package, yet a national framework for health technology assessment (HTA) has not yet been implemented. This is despite the fact that the country supported the HTA resolution at the 67th World Health Assembly (2014) requiring all countries to work towards Universal Health Coverage using HTA as a tool for priority setting. At the time of our fieldwork, the country was only piloting HTA as a tool to guide prioritisation decisions within the NHIA. So steps are being made, but the evidence advisory systems needed for particular decisions may not yet be fully formed.

In Colombia there has indeed been a recent attempt to establish a formal Health Technology Assessment body. The local body (IETS) was largely modelled on NICE in England, with key personnel from NICE involved in the establishment and governance of the body, but its institutional placement and level of influence differs considerably from the English body. IETS was not set up with a formal government mandate to make decisions for service provision in Colombia, and thus is merely advisory. The insurance based system in Colombia is also very different to the English National Health Service, and there appears to be no strong agreement on the appropriateness of using HTA metrics (like cost-effectiveness) to make decisions about services in this setting. As Chap. 9 further notes, many decisions on health service provision end up being resolved by the court system rather than the government.

Use of Routine Data to Guide Decisions

A second theme that arose in our lower and middle income settings were issues around how systems work to provide routine data to guide health sector decision making. Interestingly, the robustness of the system to use such data was not simply a reflection of the income level of the country. Indeed, it was Ethiopia that appeared to have a particularly strong emphasis on such data, building systems to use it for health sector planning. In contrast, capacity issues over data use were raised in Cambodia, along with an identified challenge in gathering data from private health providers who represent the majority of service provision in the country.

Ghana presented another case to look at how well systems of routine data align with decision structures in the country. As detailed in more depth in Chap. 4, Ghana has had investment and capacity building in its routine data system. However, that chapter further explored how such data can end up being used in an institutionalised decision making process that has strong donor influence, with international bodies playing a large role in the annual processes in which routine data are used to construct national indicators that inform the health sector plan. The analysis explored how this can result in a parallel system of evidence use and planning that was outside the normal health sector administrative hierarchy. Ethiopia, on the other hand, appeared to more strongly centrally control its planning activities, including resisting donor influence as reported in our case study.

In Germany and England, there is substantial infrastructure to collect routine data across both health systems, supported by a number of bodies created for this purpose. For a long time, data collection in England has benefited from an integrated approach applied to the NHS as a whole, with Hospital Episode Statistics being a prime example for a comprehensive and systematic approach to data collection across all hospitals in England since 1987. In Germany, such systematic data collection tends to be a more recent development, as national approaches to data collection have typically been afflicted by concerns around the privacy of personal data. In recent years, however, efforts have been made to improve the collection of routine data, for example, through the creation of the IQTiG, which is mandated with the collection of data on the quality of care across the health system.

Health-Issue Specific Decisions

In addition to deciding which health services to provide within national service packages, and the use of data to inform sector-wide planning, a third key area for evidence use in health policymaking is captured within the process of decision making within health-specific programmes. Indeed, a great deal of literature on the topic of evidence-informed policymaking in the health sector refers to how pieces of evidence can inform health issue specific decisions – such as choices between possible interventions. For example, we can see literature concerned with improving evidence use for malaria (Woelk et al. 2009), for HIV (Auerbach 2008), or for mental health decisions (Weisz et al. 2005), amongst others.

Our findings show that the institutional structures to serve these needs can be varied. Some countries will have ministerial departments that undertake research that links to other departments with specific health remits. Yet in most cases, evidence to inform decisions on health topics comes from outside Ministries of Health. This can come in the form of explicitly commissioned research dictated by, or initiated by ministry actors; or alternatively provided by external actors – be they research bodies, think tanks, international development partners, etc. – who are approaching ministry officials and departments or providing evidence of one form or another.

The use of commissioning research as a strategy relies on having resources available to do so, but also on actors to value evidence sufficient to commit them for this purpose. In many ways, research commissioning by Ministry officials may be interpreted positively as it can ensure the policy relevance of evidence generated. Yet heavy reliance on internal commissioning also risks narrowing the focus of evidence provision to those issues pre-identified or preferred by officials, potentially to the detriment of other options that have not been considered for any number of political reasons. Yet reliance on outside groups presenting information is not without challenges as well. While a much larger number of groups may provide evidence from outside official bodies, there is a risk this process is dominated by particular well-networked or well-resourced organisations, which can also direct political attention using evidence to support a given case. In our aid-dependent settings, as discussed in Chap. 10, there were concerns raised about how donor influence shapes the evidence that is created and provided to governments at times.

Arm's Length Public Health Advisory Bodies

Despite the vast differences between country settings, an institutional arrangement seen in multiple countries was the establishment of officially mandated advisory bodies that sit at 'arm's length' to the Ministry of Health. In three cases, this was explicitly a body tasked with providing advice in relation to public health: the Ethiopia Public Health Institute, the Cambodian National Institute of Public Health, and Public Health England were all mentioned as playing such roles to inform policy and practice while being placed outside of the Ministry system.

In these three cases of arm's length public health bodies, we found that they all have clear mandates to provide evidence to the decision process with appropriate linkages to do so, and in some cases their placement appeared to work well to ensure the independence of evidence advice while still remaining relevant to local needs (this was not explicitly investigated, though, in all cases). The main issue identified, however, related to capacity – with the Ethiopian and Cambodian examples showing serious limitations. In Cambodia, financial constraints were highlighted as a particular challenge. So, for example, the ability to raise salary costs by undertaking work for non-state actors was noted as a key challenge preventing the National Institute of Public Health from achieving greater potential to inform and advise the government for policymaking. In Ethiopia, the Public Health Institute also faced resource challenges, but these were presented as related to human capacity. Thus even though a directorate existed to provide policy briefs to government, only a handful were produced at the time of the fieldwork due to the limited number of staff available.

CONCLUSIONS

This chapter began by discussing the stewardship function of ministries of health, which provides them with a mandate for improving population health, but further can be seen to provide a mandate to shape the evidence advisory systems in place to inform health policy. However, when looking across a range of countries, with differing contextual features, we see a number of ways that such evidence advisory systems may function (or not) to meet the needs of health policy making. We can further identify key issues related to the ability of Ministries to serve in this stewardship role in relation to policy-relevant evidence.

In terms of authority over health policymaking itself, Ministries of Health are responsible for many key health decisions in our case study countries. Yet there are several instances where the institutional arrangements in place shift key decisions outside of direct Ministerial authority. This is perhaps most evident in Germany where the corporatist approach to governance means that actors representing the self-administration possess a good deal of authority to make decisions. As such, ministerial information sources in Germany may work in parallel with evidence systems informing the corporatist system. In Colombia, on the other hand, the Constitutional Court makes fundamental decisions on availability and provision of health services and treatments, with clear implications for evidence use given the highly technical nature of these decisions (see Chaps. 5 and 6). The judicializiation of health policy decisions in this way, takes not only decision making but also evidence advisory roles outside the control or jurisdiction of the ministry of health in that setting (Hawkins and Alvarez Rosete 2017).

Similarly, in settings in which health policy decisions were made within the legislative branch (e.g. at parliamentary level), Ministries of Health would not necessarily be involved in structuring the systems of evidence advice. Public health and health promotion decisions affecting whole populations might at times be decided at parliamentary level – for example in the UK or in Ghana. Yet there appears to be minimal involvement of ministries of health in shaping or informing the evidence advisory systems that serve the legislatures in these cases. Again, they appear to be constructed in parallel to ministry systems, or outside ministerial jurisdiction. Donor influence and control of health decisions in aid-dependent settings could lead to further cases where ministries did not have direct control over systems of evidence provision (explored more in Chap. 10).

We thus find important limitations to the idea that Ministries of Health can serve as comprehensive stewards of systems of health evidence advice, as their ability to do so will be strongly shaped by their authority and control over particular health decision types. That said, we maintain that Ministries of Health, in all case country settings, have significant roles and responsibilities for health decisions even in cases where certain key health topics are addressed in other forums or at different levels of governance. We conclude that there is a clear need for both financial and human resource capacity to ensure well-functioning evidence advisory systems serve the needs of decision makers. That said, capacity was not the only issue identified, nor were lower resources always an insurmountable challenge. Ethiopia's strength in use and control of routine data sources for planning stands out in comparison to Cambodia, which is ranks as having a marginally higher national income (World Bank 2017), but which has struggled to establish robust data management systems. Ghana has invested in its data system, but the institutional systems in place can dictate how data were subsequently used to inform health sector planning; with findings showing that routine data could end up informing planning systems greatly influenced by external donors (see Chap. 4). Even in higher income settings, we identified issues beyond those of capacity. England and Germany demonstrate a high level of scientific expertise and evidence advisory capacity, but they rely on differing mixes of systems, agencies, and bodies. The generation or synthesis of evidence through commissioned research, or through the convening of advisory groups on an *ad-hoc* basis, may reflect a positive step to ensure evidence is policy relevant, but may also lead to evidence only being provided when it is politically expedient or for issues which are already on the political agendas.

Comparing countries of varying income levels illustrates that the realm of government bodies (some at arm's length, others not) appears much more crowded in England and Germany than in our other case study countries. This may not be surprising, however, as it is possible that as institutional structures evolve over time, there will be increasing numbers of organisations, a greater division of work, and potential for higher levels of specialisation. While outside the scope of analysis here, there could be future work investigating questions around this in more depth – potentially considering levels of capacity and resource; the prominence given to evidence to inform decision; and the time and stability required to establish types of infrastructure arrangements.

While the World Health Organization has indeed identified Ministries of Health as the stewards of their population's health, decision making that shapes health outcomes may be located in a number of forums, with only some key decisions taken in Ministries of Health. However, Ministries of Health remain central to health policy decisions in all settings. We have argued here that understanding when and why policy-relevant evidence serves the needs of health decisions requires an explicitly institutional lens that can consider the structural arrangements and links between sources and providers of evidence and the relevant decision making points. Evidence can improve health decisions and outcomes, but only if it is provided in a comprehensive and timely manner to inform key decisions. Ultimately it will be the underlying structures and links of the evidence advisory systems in each country that dictate when, how, and how well this takes place.

References

[Cambodia] National Institute of Statistics Directorate for Health. 2015. *Cambodia demographic and health survey 2014.* Phnom Penh: Cambodia National Institute of Statistics Directorate for Health and ICF International.

[Germany] Federal Ministry of Health. 2015. Bundestministerum für Gesundheit. http://www.bmg.bund.de/. Accessed 5/2/2015.

African Health Observatory. 2014. Ethiopia health system: Health information, research, evidence and knowledge. http://www.aho.afro.who.int/profiles_information/index.php/Ethiopia:Health_information,_research,_evidence_and_knowledge. Accessed Sept 2016.

Alvarez-Rosete, Auturo. 2007. Modernising policy making. In *Health policy and politics*, ed. A. Hann, 41–57. Aldershot: Ashgate.

Alvarez-Rosete, Arturo. 2008. The role of the state in public health. In *International encyclopedia of public health*, ed. Kris Heggenhougen, 211–218. Oxford: Academic Press.

Auerbach, Judy. 2008. *Confronting the 'evidence' in evidence-based HIV prevention: Summary report.* San Francisco: San Francisco AIDS Foundation.

Bell, Stephen, and Andrew Hindmoor. 2009. *Rethinking governance: The centrality of the state in modern society.* Cambridge: Cambridge University Press.

Bernal, Oscar, Juan Camilo Forero, and Ian Forde. 2012. Colombia's response to crisis. *BMJ* 344: 25.

Bevir, Mark. 2010. *Democratic governance.* Princeton: Princeton University Press.

Boyle, Seán. 2011. *United Kingdom (England) health system review.* London: European Observatory on Health Systems and Policies.

Cambodia Ministry of Health. 2008. *Health strategic plan 2008–2015. Accontability, efficiency, quality, equity.* Phnom Penh: Cambodia Ministry of Health.

Castro, Hector. 2014. Assessing the feasibility of conducting and using health technology assessment in Colombia. The case of severe haemophilia. Doctor of Public Health, London School of Hygiene and Tropical Medicine.

Chalmers, Iain. 2003. Trying to do more good than harm in policy and practice: The role of rigorous, transparent, up-to-date evaluations. *The Annals of the American Academy of Political and Social Science* 589 (1): 22–40.

Chalmers, Iain, Larry V. Hedges, and Harris Cooper. 2002. A brief history of research synthesis. *Evaluation & the Health Professions* 25 (1): 12–37. https://doi.org/10.1177/0163278702025001003.

Craft, Jonathan, and Michael Howlett. 2012. Policy formulation, governance shifts and policy influence: Location and content in policy advisory systems. *Journal of Public Policy* 32 (2): 79–98.

Davies, Glyn, and Michael Keating, eds. 2000. *The future of governance.* St Leonards: Allen & Unwin.

Dodgson, Richard, Kelley Lee, Nick Drager, and World Health Organization. 2002. Global health governance: A conceptual review. London School of Hygiene and Tropical Medicine and World Health Organization.

Downie, Richard. 2016. *Sustaining improvements to public health in Ethiopia.* Washington, DC: Center for Strategic and International Studies.

Durán, Antonio, Joseph Kutzin, José M. Martin-Moreno, and Phyllida Travis. 2011. Understanding health systems: Scope, functions and objectives. In *Health systems: Health, wealth, society and wellbeing. Maidenhead, Open University Press and McGraw-Hill,* ed. Joseph Figueras and Martin McKee, 19–36. Maidenhead: Open University Press.

Ethiopia Federal Ministry of Health. 2014. *Ethiopia's fifth national health accounts, 2010/2011.* Addis Ababa: Federal Ministry of Health.

Ethiopian Academy of Science. 2013. *Report on mapping the health Reserach landscape in Ethiopia.* Addis Ababa: Ethiopian Academy of Science.

Gaym, Asheber. 2008. Health research in Ethiopia—Past, present and suggestions on the way forward. *Ethiopian Medical Journal* 46 (3): 287–308.

Hafner, Tamara, and Jeremy Shiffman. 2012. The emergence of global attention to health systems strengthening. *Health Policy and Planning* 28 (1): 41–50.

Halligan, John. 1995. Policy advice and the public service. In *Governance in a changing environment,* ed. Guy Peters and Donald J. Savoie, 138–172. Montreal: Canadian Centre for Management Development.

Hanney, Stephen, Shyama Kuruvilla, Bryony Soper, and Nicholas Mays. 2010. Who needs what from a national health research system: Lessons from reforms to the English Department of Health's R&D system. *Health Research Policy and Systems* 8 (1): 11.

Hawkins, Benjamin, and Arturo Alvarez Rosete. 2017. Judicialization and health policy in Colombia: The implications for evidence-informed policymaking. *Policy Studies Journal.* https://doi.org/10.1111/psj.12230.

Hogwood, Brian W., and Lewis A. Gunn. 1984. *Policy analysis for the real world.* Oxford: Oxford University Press.

Hustedt, Thurid, and Sylvia Veit. 2017. Policy advisory systems: Change dynamics and sources of variation. *Policy Sciences* 50 (1): 41–46.

Jones, Harry, and Camboida Economic Associate Centre for Policy Studies. 2013. *Building political ownership and technical eadership: Decision-making, political economy and knowledge use in the health sector in Cambodia.* London: Overseas Development Institute.

Kickbusch, Ilona, and David Gleicher. 2012. *Governance for health in the 21st century.* World Health Organization, Regional Office for Europe.

Kickbusch, Ilona. 2002. Perspectives on health governance in the 21st century. In Marhall Marinker and Martin Mckee (eds) *Health targets in Europe: Policy, progress and promise,* 218. London: BMJ Books.

Kjaer, Anne Mette. 2004. *Governance: Key concepts.* Cambridge: Polity Press.

———. 2011. Rhodes' contribution to governance theory: Praise, criticism and the future governance debate. *Public Administration* 89 (1): 101–113.

Kooiman, Jan. 2000. Societal governance: Levels, modes and orders of social-political interaction. In *Debating governance: Authority, steering and democracy,* ed. Jon Pierre, 138–167. Oxford: Oxford University Press.

Koon, Adam D., Krishna D. Rao, Nhan T. Tran, and Abdul Ghaffar. 2013. Embedding health policy and systems research into decision-making processes in low-and middle-income countries. *BMC Health Research Policy and Systems* 11 (1): 30.

LaRocca, Rebecca, Jennifer Yost, Maureen Dobbins, Donna Ciliska, and Michelle Butt. 2012. The effectiveness of knowledge translation strategies used in public health: A systematic review. *BMC Public Health* 12 (1): 751.

Lavis, John N., G. Emmanuel Guindon, David Cameron, Boungnong Boupha, Masoumeh Dejman, Eric J. Osei, and Ritu Sadana. 2010. Bridging the gaps between research, policy and practice in low- and middle-income countries: A survey of researchers. *CMAJ.* https://doi.org/10.1503/cmaj.081164.

Lewis, Richard, Arturo Alvarez-Rosete, and Nicholas Mays. 2006. *How to regulate health care in England? An international perspective*: King's Fund.

McQueen, David, Matthias Wismar, Vivian Lin, Catherine M. Jones, and Maggie Davies, eds. 2012. *Intersectoral governance for health in all policies. Structures, actions and experiences.* Malta: World Health Organization on behalf of the European Observatory on Health Systems and Policies.

NICE. 2017. NICE Charter. National Institute for Health and Care Excellence. https://www.nice.org.uk/media/default/about/who-we-are/nice_charter.pdf

Nutley, Sandra M., Isabel Walter, and Huw T.O. Davies. 2007. *Using evidence: How research can inform public services.* Bristol: The Policy Press.
Parkhurst, Justin. 2017. *The politics of evidence: From evidence based policy to the good governance of evidence.* Abingdon: Routledge.
Piere, Jan, and B. Guy Peters. 2000. *Governance, politics and the state.* Basingstoke: Macmillian.
Pierre, Jon. 2000. *Debating governance: Authority, steering and democracy.* Oxford: Oxford University Press.
Reich, Michael R. 2002. Reshaping the state from above, from within, from below: Implications for public health. *Social Science & Medicine* 54 (11): 1669–1675.
Rhodes, Roderick Arthur William. 1996. The new governance: Governing without government. *Political studies* 44 (4): 652–667.
Rhodes, Rod A.W. 1997. *Understanding governance: Policy networks, governance, reflexivity and accountability.* Philadelphia: Open University Press.
Richards, David, and Martin J. Smith. 2002. *Governance and public policy in the UK.* Oxford: Oxford University Press.
Rosenau, James N. 1995. Governance in the twenty-first century. *Global Governance* 1 (1): 13–43.
Saltman, Richard B., and Odile Ferroussier-Davis. 2000. The concept of stewardship in health policy. *Bulletin of the World Health Organization* 78 (6): 732–739.
Saltman, Richard B., Antonio Durán, and Hans F.W. Dubois. 2011. *Governing public hospitals. Reform strategies and the movement towards institutional autonomy.* Copenhagen: European Observatory on Health Systems and Policy, WHO Regional Office for Europe.
Shaw, Sara E., Jill Russell, Trisha Greenhalgh, and Maja Korica. 2014. Thinking about think tanks in health care: A call for a new research agenda. *Sociology of Health & Illness* 36 (3): 447–461.
Shergold, Miriam, and Jonathan Grant. 2008. Freedom and need: The evolution of public strategy for biomedical and health research in England. *Health Research Policy and Systems* 6 (1): 2.
Stoker, Gerry. 1998. Governance as theory: Five propositions. *International Social Science Journal* 50 (155): 17–28.
UK Government. 2013. *What works: Evidence centres for social policy.* London: UK Cabinet Office.
van Kammen, Jessika, Don de Savigny, and Nelson Sewankambo. 2006. Using knowledge brokering to promote evidence-based policy-making: The need for support structures. *Bulletin of the World Health Organization* 84: 608–612.
Weisz, John R., Irwin N. Sandler, Joseph A. Durlak, and Barry S. Anton. 2005. Promoting and protecting youth mental health through evidence-based prevention and treatment. *American Psychologist* 60 (6): 628.

WHO. 2000. *The world health report 2000 – Health systems: Improving performance*. Geneva: World Health Organization.

———. 2003. *The world health report 2003. Shaping the future*. Geneva: World Health Organization.

———. 2007. *Everybody's business. Strengthening health systems to improve health outcomes. WHO's framework for action*. Geneva: World Health Organization.

———. 2008. *Primary care. Now more than ever*. Geneva: World Health Organization.

WHOROE. 2008. *Tallinn charter on health systems, health and wealth*. Copenhagen: WHO Regional Office for Europe.

Woelk, Godfrey, Karen Daniels, Julie Cliff, Simon Lewin, Esperança Sevene, Benedita Fernandes, Alda Mariano, Sheillah Matinhure, Andrew D. Oxman, and John N. Lavis. 2009. Translating research into policy: Lessons learned from eclampsia treatment and malaria control in three southern African countries. *Health Research Policy and Systems* 7 (31): 1–14.

World Bank. 2011. *Cambodia – More efficient government spending for strong and inclusive growth: Integrated fiduciary assessment and public expenditure review (IFPER)*. Phnom Penh: The World Bank.

———. 2017. World development indicators database. http://databank.worldbank.org/data/download/GNIPC.pdf

Yamin, Alicia Ely, and Oscar Parra-Vera. 2010. Judicial protection of the right to health in Colombia: From social demands to individual claims to public debates. *Hastings International & Comparative Law Review* 33: 431.

Open Access   This chapter is licensed under the terms of the Creative Commons Attribution 4.0 International License (http://creativecommons.org/licenses/by/4.0/), which permits use, sharing, adaptation, distribution and reproduction in any medium or format, as long as you give appropriate credit to the original author(s) and the source, provide a link to the Creative Commons license and indicate if changes were made.

The images or other third party material in this chapter are included in the chapter's Creative Commons license, unless indicated otherwise in a credit line to the material. If material is not included in the chapter's Creative Commons license and your intended use is not permitted by statutory regulation or exceeds the permitted use, you will need to obtain permission directly from the copyright holder.

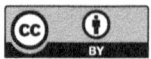

CHAPTER 9

Evidence Use and the Institutions of the State: The Role of Parliament and the Judiciary

Stefanie Ettelt

INTRODUCTION

Most analyses of the role of scientific evidence in health policy see health system governance as predominantly the responsibility of the Government, with the Ministry of Health being its main representative. The World Health Organization (WHO), for example, emphasised the steering role of ministries in improving health and health system performance (Travis et al. 2002). Yet what is sometimes overlooked is that ministries operate in context, with other state institutions interacting and shaping its role. The Ministry of Health may be the main actor responsible for health within the executive, but it operates within a larger institutional context, i.e. the 'political system'. This definition by Scott and Mcloughlin emphasises the interaction of formal and informal institutions that shape the plethora of political processes, roles and responsibilities that together form the state:

S. Ettelt (✉)
London School of Hygiene and Tropical Medicine, London, UK
e-mail: stefanie.ettelt@lshtm.ac.uk

Political systems are the formal and informal political processes by which decisions are made concerning the use, production and distribution of resources in any given society. Formal political institutions can determine the process for electing leaders; the roles and responsibilities of the executive and legislature; the organisation of political representation (through political parties); and the accountability and oversight of the state. Informal and customary political systems, norms and rules can operate within or alongside these formal political institutions. (Scott and Mcloughlin 2014: n.p.)

This chapter examines the role of two of the institutions of the state that influence health policymaking and health system governance in addition to government. With health policy we mean all national or subnational policies that have an intentional bearing on population health and health care provision; health system governance refers to the steering of the health system with all its components. These definitions overlap, as they should, but as not all health policies relate to health system governance and not all governance decisions may be considered policies.

The chapter concentrates on the legislature and the judiciary, which are typically anchored in constitutional law (the United Kingdom is the example in which constitutional rules are in existence but are "unwritten"). Therefore, this chapter will examine the role of (1) parliaments in making legislation and scrutinising the actions of government, and (2) the legal system, forming the judiciary and its role in arbitrating conflicts between policy actors and in scrutinising the compatibility of decisions by government and parliament with existing law.

Understanding the role of the legislative and judiciary is important to contextualise the role of health ministries analysed in earlier chapters and their approach to making use of research evidence to inform decisions. The chapter takes the observation as a starting point that other bodies of 'the state' are often involved in the policy process and should therefore be considered relevant when we analyse the role of scientific evidence in health policymaking. Yet the constellation of these bodies varies between countries as they reflect differences in political systems, which translates into significant differences in how health policymaking and health system governance are influenced by them.

The chapter does not attempt to cover all bodies of the state relevant to health policy or all aspects of each country's political system. Instead, it aims to provide a broad overview by extracting relevant examples from the case studies of the GRIP-Health project and reflect on similarities and differences between them. There are few empirical studies of how evidence from research is incorporated in decision making processes within parliaments and courts (two of them included in this book), or if there are any, they are dispersed between different academic disciplines and not fully explored from the perspective of evidence-based policy-making. This chapter wants to highlight this gap by drawing attention to the relevance of legislators and courts in using evidence to exercise their mandate. It primarily does so by exploring the use of evidence in relation to their function of holding government to account, which has the benefit of allowing us to reflect on the checks and balances on governmental power and the limits of its decision-making relating to health policy.

INSTITUTIONS OF THE STATE AND THEIR ROLE IN USING EVIDENCE FOR HEALTH POLICY-MAKING

It is sometimes assumed that health policymaking largely takes place in central government, with ministries of health being the only state actors. Indeed, the WHO, highlighting the need for stewardship in health system governance, largely called on ministries of health to become responsible 'stewards' in driving health policy development and system reform (Travis et al. 2002). There are multiple critiques of this assumption, for example, with regard to countries in which responsibility for health are shared between different levels of government (Ettelt et al. 2010). This exists in many forms, for example in federalist countries in which responsibility for health policy is shared by different levels of government (Banting and Corbett 2001). But even among countries that are not federalist in the sense that they consist of a federation of states with separate state governments and parliaments, there is much variation with regard to the distribution of responsibility for health and the health system (Saltman et al. 2007). The United Kingdom with its four countries – England, Scotland, Wales and the Northern Ireland – is a case in point, as each country has its own health department and National Health Service, with only a few functions (e.g. emergency response) being centralised.

In addition, in many countries the decision-making power for health policymaking is also diffused among the institutions of the state, especially parliament and the judiciary. This particularly emphasises the role of national law, both in terms of making and in interpreting legislation, in health policy-making and system governance. The countries selected for this study cover different political regime types (ranging from democratic to non-democratic) and different constitutional structures (e.g. unitary vs. federal states; degree of executive control) (Ettelt et al. 2016). The comparison of political systems of the six countries selected for this study highlights three important differences:

- First, in some countries, the health policy and system governance function is highly centralised with the ministry of health being the main, and sometimes only player, with parliament and the judiciary being less influential. Ethiopia, Cambodia and Ghana broadly fall into this category for reasons that include both constitutional separation of power and practices of collaborative deliberation. In Ghana, for instance, in theory, parliament should approve the sectoral budgets for any financial year and coordinate its decision with the Ministry of Health responsible for the internal evaluation of the performance of the health system and its policies. Yet coordination does not happen in practice; while both processes tend to happen simultaneously, there is little overlap of the personnel involved in each and hence the coordination between both processes is limited. In Germany, in contrast, health system governance is almost entirely devolved to corporatist actors operating within a legal framework developed by the Federal Parliament, with the Federal Ministry of Health being only responsible for a relatively narrowly defined set of policy decisions and accountability functions (Ettelt et al. 2010).
- The second difference relates to the role of parliament in making health policy decisions and in scrutinising government actions in relation to policy development and health system governance. While parliament has some role in health policymaking in most countries, by way of debating, developing and eventually passing legislation, there are substantial differences in the extent to which parliament uses its powers to scrutinize government policy both ex ante and ex post, and the extent this scrutiny involves questioning the type of knowledge used to inform its decisions including scientific evidence.
- A third difference relates to the role of the judiciary in health policy and health system governance. Colombia and Germany stand out among the selected countries in this respect as in both countries the judiciary has a strong role in challenging the decisions of government and other health policy actors (e.g. the corporatist self-administration). The right to challenge these decisions in the courts is inscribed in constitutional law, which define both the balance of power within the state and the scope for action by citizens and others (e.g. provider organisations,

insurers, corporatist actors) to defend their rights in case of violation. In other countries, in contrast, the judiciary is more restrained in intervening in government decisions either because of customary authority given to the government (in England) or because the judiciary is not sufficiently independent from those ruling in government (in Cambodia).

In the following two sections the role of the legislature and the judiciary and their potential for evidence use will be investigated in more detail, starting with the role of parliaments.

LEGISLATURES: THE ROLE OF PARLIAMENTS

Given their constitutional role, parliaments should have a major influence on evidence use in health system governance and health policies. However, whether this happens in practice is an empirical question and this question has not yet been much researched.

In principle, there are (at least) two roles for parliament that can create opportunities for evidence use. The first role is to develop legislation and to set the legislative framework for health system governance. This includes initiating major health care reform (e.g. setting up the current system of health care financing in Colombia), but can also involve a broad spectrum of legislation that applies to any aspect of health care financing and delivery, health promotion, and preventative and public health measures (as discussed e.g. in the chapter on Ghana). Such decisions would warrant good information, hence there is a potential role for research evidence to influence these processes (constituting some form of 'instrumental' use).

The second role is for parliament to hold government to account for its decisions and actions. This can include both the use of scientific studies as a means to exercise accountability (e.g. evaluation of government policies or analyses of health system monitoring data) and the requirement of government and its constituent parts to demonstrate that decisions are well founded, which may include considerations of supporting evidence from research.

The analysis of the countries selected in this book suggests that there is great variation in the role of parliament in using, and enforcing, evidence use in health policymaking. Crucially, parliaments vary in their involvement in health policymaking, but also in the extent to which they hold government to account. In some countries, as outlined above, health policymaking and health system governance are mostly the domain of the executive with parliamentary involvement and oversight being limited or non-existent (Newman et al. 2013). In other countries, parliaments decide on a wide range of health policies and health system governance issues. As an example, Parliaments in England and Ghana both approve the budget allocation for health care. The Federal Parliament in Germany (composed of the Federal Assembly (*Bundestag*) and the Federal Council (*Bundesrat*)), in contrast, does not have authority over the budget, as this is held jointly by sickness funds as funds are collected through a social insurance system. Yet in Germany, the Federal Parliament plays a crucial role in setting, and monitoring, contribution rates to social health insurance thus influencing the ability of sickness funds to increase the budget significantly.

The analysis of the country case studies suggests that there is great variation as to the role of parliament in using, and enforcing, evidence use in health policymaking. Overall the verdict is not positive. In our study, examples of parliaments or parliamentarians engaging with research and opportunities for using evidence to come to better informed decisions were few and far between, particular with regard to informing legislative decisions. The analysis of minimum volumes policy in Germany (aimed at improving outcomes of complex interventions in hospitals) is a case in point. Parliament seemed not to have engaged with any evidence, despite the fact that the policy proposal was inspired by findings from health services research. Yet the scientific evidence base for minimum volumes became a major cause of disagreement at later stages of the policy process, including in the courts. In Germany, both chambers of Parliament are supported by an in-house scientific service, but its role is largely invisible to the public (it briefly surfaced in a recent scandal where a minister had used the service to co-write his PhD (Blechschmidt et al. 2011)). A recent study on the role of research in the UK Parliament, conducted by researchers of the Parliamentary Office of Science and Technology, concluded that almost all Members of Parliament and their staff participating in the survey (83 out of a total of 85) found research evidence useful for their work. However, most respondents applied a wide definition of what they meant by 'research' and 'evidence', including scientific research as well as other forms of research and knowledge (Kenny et al. 2017).

Countries also vary in whether health policy is mostly made through legislation, like in Germany and Colombia, or whether decisions relating to health policy and health system governance are mostly made through government decree and secondary legislation. Colombia's bicameral Parliament (the Congress) plays a substantial role in health system governance as most aspects of health policy are based on primary legislation (although there is also the possibility of a presidential decree). When the current system of health care financing was created through 'Law 100' in 1993 it was expected that much of the detailed principles that are required for its full implementation would be developed by subsequent legislatures. However, this has proven to be a slow process with the Congress having difficulties in forming sustainable majorities to make substantial decisions over a longer period of time as required for the implementation of Law 100.

Weyrauch et al. (2016) note that political parties can play a prominent role in channelling scientific evidence to inform legislation. However, in Colombia, to stay with the example, Parliament has a reputation for being fragmented and its members tend not to vote along party lines. Political parties are deemed weak and "lack[ing] the coherence and stability needed to effectively make policy" (Pachón and Johnson 2016: 73). This tendency to fragmentation in consequence allows the Government to exercise power over Parliament and orchestrate legislative action. Pachon and Johnson (2016) note that bills brought forward by the Government have a much higher chance to be turned into legislation than bills promoted by members of parliament, suggesting that the Government has substantial influence over the legislative process, for example by influencing the selection of chairs and rapporteurs on parliamentary committees.

In our case study on Colombia, Alvarez-Rosete and Hawkins (in this book) demonstrate that legislation is often justified by reference to scientific evidence and it is possible that committees engage with studies relating to relevant topics. However, it is difficult to see what incentives members of parliament might have to use evidence or scrutinise the Government's use of evidence. Dargent (2015) also noted that, in Colombia, Ministry of Health officials hold most technical expertise and have often play a pivotal role in informing the development of health legislation, again tipping the balance in favour of government.

One condition for parliaments to exercise their function to oversee governments is that the legislature has a degree of independence from the executive. Arguably, this is inherently difficult in parliamentary systems in which the executive is formed by majority holders elected into parliament. However, the question is whether parliament is sufficiently separate from government so that members of parliament see it as their collective responsibility to hold their government to account. If this is not the case, for example where both government and parliament are dominated by the same group of people (as in Cambodia), it is unlikely that parliament is in a position to review and challenge government actions.

Parliaments can also be limited in their capacity to scrutinise proposals from the executive, which produces the vast amount of legislative initiatives. In Ghana, the Select Committee on Health can initiate inquiries on health policy matters to hold the Government to account, but its efforts are constrained by its limited budgetary and professional capacity.

Lindberg (2010) notes that Parliamentary scrutiny of government policy in Ghana was high in the years 1997–2000 (the second presidential term of Jerry John Rawlings in the Fourth Republic), with subsequent parliaments being less active in challenging government action. The problem Lindberg diagnoses is that members of parliament are themselves not held to account by their constituents for their role in scrutinising government, but are rewarded, and kept in post, for their ability to secure resources for local projects and investments. Access to such resources is controlled by the Government which therefore can reward (or penalise) members of parliament for their support (or the lack of it) for government decisions. Mechanisms such as questions to the Government from the floor are possible, but they are more likely to be used to inquire about progress in the implementation of local projects than about policies relevant to the populace as a whole (Lindberg 2010). With the accountability function being ineffective, the ability of parliament – while democratically elected and thriving in this respect – to scrutinise government is weak. This weakness is compounded by a lack of resources and capacity of parliamentary services.

The importance of accountability mechanisms for evidence use is also highlighted by the role of the Parliament (composed of the House of Commons and the House of Lords) in the UK. The UK Parliament passes primary legislation relating to health, which provides the framework for the National Health Service (NHS), public health and other health-related policies. It also scrutinises health policy that the Government develops and implements via secondary legislation through its Department of Health. A number of mechanisms are available for this purpose, including parliamentary debates, and questions put to ministers, the department and posed directly to the Prime Minister. Evidence from research may play a part in these mechanisms (Kenny et al. 2017), yet its use is highly variable, topic dependent and often superseded by debates about the worthiness of policy goals in the first place. The debate about the controversial 2012 health care reform is a case in point, in which Members of Parliament challenged the intention of the Government to privatise the NHS much more forcefully than they demanded the existence of any studies in support of the proposal for large-scale restructuring and the strengthening of provider competition (Timmins 2012). The Government was criticised for not using evidence, but this critique came from actors outside the legislature, such as policy think tanks (IoG 2012).

Both the House of Commons and the House of Lords are supported in their work by research and library services, however, the extent to which these information services are used and are seen as relevant by members is highly variable. In contrast, scientific evidence is often central in the work of the Health Select Committee. In the 2015–17 Parliamentary term, the Committee conducted 24 inquiries on topics as wide ranging as the state of the NHS finances, the Government's actions on suicide prevention, the effects of Brexit on health and social care services, and the state of public health after the restructuring of the sector in 2013. The Committee invites public sector and civil society organisations to make submissions for a topic, which are often bolstered by substantial references to studies. It also invites a broad range of experts, including researchers, to give evidence before the committee. After deliberating the evidence from all sources (scientific or not), the committee publishes its verdict in a report available from its website (e.g. HoC 2016). However, the extent to which UK Select Committees are able to hold the Government to account is debated. King and Crewe (2013: 355), in their book "The blunders of our Governments", argue that such committees "seldom seek to delve deeply into the origins of policies as distinct from their merits and generally fight shy of addressing issues that already are, or might become, issues of partisan controversy".

THE JUDICIARY: THE ROLE OF COURTS

The judiciary – often referred to as the third power of the state – applies and interprets the law of a country in the name of the state. Countries vary in whether the judiciary can have a role in developing legislation, either through commenting, or even approving, proposed bills or through setting precedence that informs future decisions of courts.

This function is represented, for example, by the Constitutional Court in Colombia, which has authority, as per the Colombian constitution, to review legislation passed by the Congress if the bill affects constitutional rights (Hernández Álvarez 2013). The Constitutional Court can also decide to step in if it finds that legislative and executive bodies have failed to act. This has created a dynamic in which political actors tend to defer to the Court for resolution on contested issues that they are unable to resolve by other means.

The judiciary can also have a role in holding the government and parliament to account, for example through the mechanisms of constitutional complaint or judicial review. In Germany, the Federal Government and Parliament tend to consult senior judges at the German Constitutional Court on policies that affect constitutional rights to avoid a retrospective "complaint of unconstitutionality" (*Verfassungsklage*) that can result in legislation being revoked and returned to legislators (Landfried 1994). There is no suggestion that courts are particularly interested or indeed equipped to advise other state bodies about matters of scientific evidence, as advice will be focused on aspects of legality and couched in legal terms only. However, depending on the issue in question it is possible that studies play a role in legal argumentation in case of review (as demonstrated in the chapter on minimum volumes in this book).

However, it is not a given that courts are in a position to challenge governments as this (as with parliament) requires a good degree of independence between the executive and the judiciary. Courts can also arbitrate in conflicts between individuals and organisations, often using a broad spectrum of law that has a bearing on health and health policy (e.g. medical law; social law; criminal law, administrative law). In some countries, courts play a prominent role in arbitrating access to care decisions, especially those that provide a constitutional right to health or health care (e.g. Colombia, Germany). These decisions typically cut across litigation on behalf of individuals (i.e. patients, members of sickness funds) and the politico-administrative system mandated with making decisions about collective health service coverage (for example through bodies such as the National Institute For Health and Care Excellence (NICE) in England or the Institute for Health Technology Assessment (IETS) in Colombia).

Such litigation is widespread in Colombia, where a constitutional right to health provides the legal basis for patients to challenge decisions by insurers if these deny funding treatments. Between 1999 and 2014 over 1.3 million right-to-health cases were brought to the Constitutional Court (Defensoría del Pueblo 2015). Such court cases draw on the legal instrument of 'tutelas' which are "informal and expedite injunctions that allow citizens to seek judicial protection when their basic rights are threatened by the state or by a third party" (Lamprea 2014: 133). The court therefore has the power to reverse a decision made by insurers, both public and private, as well as decisions made by IETS, even if these decisions have been based on rigorous health technology assessment. This is problematic, as the right to health is interpreted in a way that allows individuals to have access to (government-funded) treatment even if this treatment is proven to be ineffective or excessively costly.

Pharmaceutical companies have latched on this opportunity and have made a business model of providing legal support to patients to gain additional funding. However, while the behaviour of the court has been decried as inappropriately interventionist, it has also been argued that this is the only route that patients can take to challenge the decisions of insurers. The argument is that the Ministry of Health has been unable to effectively regulate and police the behaviour of insurers and the price setting of pharmaceutical companies that both could help to ease pressure on courts. Lamprea (2014: 158) therefore suggests that the Constitutional Court in Colombia acts like the proverbial "canary in the coal mine that signals deeper institutional dysfunctions within Colombia's health sector".

Courts in Germany have a prominent role in access to treatment decisions, but in contrast to Colombia most cases are dealt with by Social Courts (i.e. a system of courts concerned with social security matters) rather than the Federal Constitutional Court. In 2005, the Constitutional Court laid down rules for applying the constitutional 'right to life' included in the German Basic Law (which expands to a right to health care). This decision provides the basis for the decisions of all courts to which these rules apply, forcing sickness funds to reimburse treatment, including in cases in which evidence of effectiveness was absent or highly questionable (Ettelt in press). However, compared with Colombia, the caseload in Germany is relatively modest, with less than 400 cases between 2005 and the end of 2015 (RUB 2016).

In contrast, courts play a much more limited role in treatment decisions in England, where no constitutional right to health exists. Since the inception of NICE, there have been less than a handful of cases in which NHS patients sought legal redress against decisions by NICE to withhold (or, more precisely, not mandate local NHS organisations to provide) treatment in the NHS. Littlejohns et al. (2012) noted that there is only a narrowly defined set of reasons that patients can employ to take NICE, or any Government agency, to court. These reasons are that NICE has exceeded its mandate (defined by Parliament and the Secretary of State for Health), that the institute acted unfairly or that the decision cannot be 'reasonably' justified, all of which can be refuted by reference to mandate and procedure, which can include reference to appropriate use to scientific evidence (also Syrett 2010).

However, more recently, there were a number of cases of patients who took NHS England (the central governance body overseeing the NHS) to court for rejecting applications for treatment funding. In May 2016, the High Court ordered NHS England to provide a teenager with narcolepsy with the requested drug at least for three months, in spite of NHS England not considering the drug as sufficiently cost-effective (HSJ 2016). The court ruled that the case met the criteria of "exceptionality" and judged that the reasoning of NHS England was "unsupportable". Yet such legal challenges to treatment decisions of NHS governing bodies that are effectively government agencies are considered unusual and undesirable, as it is argued that courts should not become involved in decisions about resource allocation. Such decisions should be made by government and related administrative bodies (Ford and Tracy 2016).

In interviews, conducted in Cambodia, Ghana and Ethiopia the judiciary was not mentioned as an institutional actor that impacts on health policy or health system governance decisions. This may be a reflection of our interview strategy but it also resonates with our observation of the unstable or emerging role of the judiciary in these countries and/or a lack of judicial independence that does not allow courts to challenge the government. Cambodia, for example, only begun (re-)building its judicial system after democratisation in 1993 following several decades with no legal system in place. However, the judiciary is institutionally weak and dominated by the interests of the ruling elite which also dominate the executive and legislature (Dressel 2014; McCarthy and Un 2015). There is therefore no mechanism through which the judiciary could hold the government to account (with the trial against former Khmer Rouge leaders being a potential exception) and courts are unlikely to be involved in health policy decisions.

THE INSTITUTIONS OF THE STATE MATTER FOR THE STUDY OF EVIDENCE USE IN HEALTH POLICY AND HEALTH SYSTEM GOVERNANCE

This chapter has discussed a number of examples from our programme of work that illustrate how the design and functioning of state institutions can shape the accountability mechanism between the government, parliament and the judiciary and the different places in which decision-making in relation to health policy and health system making can happen at the national level. While ministries of health are the pivotal (if not only) actors in health policymaking, their role is highly dependent on the institutional configuration of the state.

Our country case studies showed a variety of such constellations, particularly focusing on parliament (legislature) and courts (judiciary), their role in scrutinising government policy and their involvement in decision making relating to health policy. While there are few studies specifically examining the role of evidence use in decisions in parliaments or the judiciary this chapter wants to shine a spotlight on the fact that these institutions often have a role in health policymaking and health system governance which should not be overlooked.

The chapter hints at a number of tensions between decision-making structures and demands for better use of research evidence in policy-making.

Parliament provides a key mechanism for holding government to account, however, this is not a given and in many situations this is not sufficiently exercised. There are many reasons why parliaments can find it difficult to hold governments to account, although these are likely to vary greatly. It also can be argued that attention of parliament for government activities, in health or elsewhere, is likely to be sporadic and incomplete, and depended on the interests, qualification and attention span of their members. However, in countries in which the parliament (often through committees) uses evidence and demands evidence use from the government, this can provide a powerful stimulus for better evidence use throughout the sector.

There are only a few examples of courts being involved in health policy decisions within the scope of this book. Examples of court involvement in access to treatment decisions in Germany and Colombia show that the relationship can be complicated with courts likely to give preference to constitutional principles that emphasise individual rights over concerns about effectiveness or affordability. However, different judicial practices in different countries have brought about a variety of approaches that may or may not include an assessment of evidence from studies. Courts can also have a place in reviewing Government policies through mechanisms such as judicial review or 'constitutional challenge', although the effect of evidence use is unclear.

REFERENCES

Banting, K.G., and S.M. Corbett. 2001. *Health policy and federalism: A comparative perspective on multi-level governance.* Kingston: Institute of Intergovernmental Relations, Queen's University.

Blechschmidt, P., T. Schultz, and R. Preuß. 2011. Guttenberg helped himself to six Bundestag reports [Guttenberg bediente sich bei sechs Bundestags-Expertisen], Süddeutsche Zeitung, February 25.

Dargent, E. 2015. *Technocracy and democracy in Latin America: The experts running government.* Cambridge: Cambridge University Press.

Defensoría del Pueblo. 2015. La Tutela y los Derechos a la Salud y a la Seguridad Social [The tutela and the right to health and the social security]. Bogota: Defensoría del Pueblo de Colombia.
Dressel, B. 2014. Governance, courts and politics in Asia. *Journal of Contemporary Asia* 44 (2): 259–278.
Ettelt, S. in press. Access to treatment and the constitutional right to health in Germany: A triumph of hope over evidence? *Health Economics, Policy, and Law*.
Ettelt, S., N. Mays, K. Chevreul, A. Nikolentzos, S. Thomson, and E. Nolte. 2010. Involvement of ministries of health in health service coverage decisions: Is England an aberrant case? *Social Policy and Administration* 44 (3): 225–243.
Ettelt, S., B. Hawkins, and A. Alvarez-Rosete. 2016. Analysing evidence use in national health policy-making – An institutional approach. http://blogs.lshtm. ac.uk/griphealth/files/2016/09/Analysing-evidence-use-in-national-health-policy-making-an-institutional-approach.pdf. Accessed 15 Nov 2017.
Ford, G., and J. Tracy. 2016. Judicial review update: NHS England ordered to fund treatment. Hempsons (Lawyers), London, July 22. http://www. hempsons.co.uk/news/judicial-review-update-nhs-england-ordered-fund-treatment. Accessed 26 Oct 2016.
Hernández Álvarez, M. 2013. Ley Estatutaria debe superar el debate tecnócrata. *Un periódico* 166 (6).
HoC. 2016. Public health post-2013. Second report of session 2016–17. London: House of Commons Health Committee.
HSJ. 2016. Third time lucky for NHS England? *HSJ*, 3 August 2016.
IoG. 2012. *Learning the lessons from 'never again'?* London: Institute for Government.
Kenny, C., D.C. Rose, A. Hobbs, C. Tyler, and J. Blackstock. 2017. *The role of research in the UK parliament. Volume one*. London: Houses of Parliament.
King, A., and I. Crewe. 2013. *The blunders of our governments*. London: Oneworld.
Lamprea, E. 2014. Colombia's right-to-health litigation in the context of health care reform. In *The right to health at the public/private divide. A global comparative study*, ed. C.M. Flood and A. Gross, 131–158. Cambridge: Cambridge University Press.
Landfried, C. 1994. The judicialization of politics in Germany. *International Political Science Review* 15 (2): 113–124.
Lindberg, S.I. 2010. What accountability pressure do MPs in Africa face and how do they respond? Evidence from Ghana. *Journal of Modern African Studies* 48 (1): 117–142.
Littlejohns, P., T. Sharma, and K. Jeong. 2012. Social values and health priority setting in England: "Values" based decision making. *Journal of Health Organization and Management* 26 (3): 363–371.
McCarthy, S., and K. Un. 2015. The evolution of rule of law in Cambodia. Democratization, Published online December 28. http://www.tandfonline. com/doi/full/10.1080/13510347.2015.1103736

Newman, K., A. Capillo, A. Famurewa, C. Nath, and W. Siyanbola. 2013. What is the evidence on evidence-informed policy making? In *Lessons from the International Conference on Evidence-Informed Policy Making*. Oxford: International Network for the Availability of Scientific Publications.
Pachón, M., and B.B. Johnson. 2016. When's the party (or coalition)? Agenda-setting in a highly fragmented, decentralized legislature. *Journal of Politics in Latin America* 8 (2): 71–100.
RUB. 2016. Nikolaus project. Overview of decisions [Nikolaus-Projekt. Übersicht der Entscheidungen]. Ruhr-Universität Bochum. http://nikolaus-beschluss.de/decisions. Accessed 12 Nov 2016.
Saltman, R.B., V. Bankauskaite, and K. Vrangbæk, eds. 2007. *Decentralization in health care. Strategies and outcome*. Maidenhead: Open University Press.
Scott, Z., and C. Mcloughlin. 2014. *Political systems: Topic guide*. Birmingham: GSDRC, University of Birmingham.
Syrett, K. 2010. Health technology appraisal and the courts: Accountability for reasonableness and the judicial model of procedural justice. *Health Economics, Policy and Law* 6 (4): 469–488.
Timmins, N. 2012. *Never again? The story of the health and social care act 2012*. London: The King's Fund and Institute for Government.
Travis, P., D. Egger, P. Davies, and A. Mechbal. 2002. *Towards better stewardship: Concepts and critical issues*. Geneva: World Health Organization.
Weyrauch, V., L. Echt, and S. Suliman. 2016. *Knowledge into policy: Going beyond 'context matters'*. Oxford: INASP.

Open Access This chapter is licensed under the terms of the Creative Commons Attribution 4.0 International License (http://creativecommons.org/licenses/by/4.0/), which permits use, sharing, adaptation, distribution and reproduction in any medium or format, as long as you give appropriate credit to the original author(s) and the source, provide a link to the Creative Commons license and indicate if changes were made.

The images or other third party material in this chapter are included in the chapter's Creative Commons license, unless indicated otherwise in a credit line to the material. If material is not included in the chapter's Creative Commons license and your intended use is not permitted by statutory regulation or exceeds the permitted use, you will need to obtain permission directly from the copyright holder.

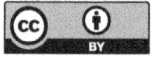

CHAPTER 10

Evidence and Policy in Aid-Dependent Settings

Justin Parkhurst, Siobhan Leir, Helen Walls, Elisa Vecchione, and Marco Liverani

INTRODUCTION

As has been noted in earlier chapters of this book, comparative institutional analyses can be particularly difficult when national contexts differ widely. As such, identifying common features in the political or institutional contexts across different settings can be important. One highly relevant contextual feature that is shared across a range of lower income settings is the presence, and potential influence, of international donor

J. Parkhurst (✉)
London School of Economics and Political Science, London, UK
e-mail: j.parkhurst@lse.ac.uk

S. Leir • H. Walls • E. Vecchione • M. Liverani
London School of Hygiene and Tropical Medicine, London, UK
e-mail: siobhan.leir@lshtm.ac.uk; helen.walls@lshtm.ac.uk; e.vecchione@ucl.ac.uk; marco.liverani@lshtm.ac.uk

© The Author(s) 2018
J. Parkhurst et al. (eds.), *Evidence Use in Health Policy Making*, International Series on Public Policy, https://doi.org/10.1007/978-3-319-93467-9_10

agencies (or 'aid' agencies) that provide funding and assistance to recipient governments (often classified as 'Official Development Assistance' or ODA). Of course, there are a wide variety of aid modalities and relationships with these agencies in recipient country settings. International donors can be bilateral or multilateral in their orientation (i.e. representing specific governments or collections of countries); they may be private philanthropic (e.g. foundations like the Rockefeller Foundation or Bill and Melinda Gates Foundation); or issue-specific aid mechanisms (e.g. the Global Fund to fight AIDS, Tuberculosis and Malaria; or Gavi – the Vaccine Alliance).

In many parts of the world, aid provision and donor relationships have been seen to have historical strategic and political origins (Van Belle 2004). Lancaster (2008), for instance, argues that most aid – particularly from the US – originated out of cold war diplomacy. While McDougall (2011) argues that Australia's aid programme has aimed to improve security in the pacific region. Yet while each country's arrangements, and historical engagement, with donors will have its own unique features, for comparative analyses it can be a useful starting point to consider shared experiences involved when outside agencies provide financial support for social policies and public services in recipient countries. The role of donors in the use of evidence to inform health policy was thus identified as a theme in three of the GRIP-Health programme case study countries, Cambodia, Ethiopia, and Ghana, where levels of donor assistance (in terms of net Official Development Assistance) were, respectively, 5.1%, 6.5%, and 3.0% of gross national income, at the time of our research (according to 2014 World Bank estimates (World Bank)).

Concerns have been raised, particularly in the international development literature, about the influence that donors may have over domestic policy agendas, policy decisions, and governance arrangements through the aid relationship. Development scholars have often taken a critical stance towards conditionality attached to aid and policy-based lending, in part for its imposition on the sovereignty of recipient countries to make their own policy choices (c.f. Koeberle 2003; Mosley et al. 1995). In the health sector, for instance, Okuonzi and Macrae (1995) ask the fundamental question of 'whose policy is it anyway?' to challenge the influence donors had over priority setting in health in Uganda. Outside the specific confines of health, Chabal (1992) has argued that:

> Aid has become an integral part of state policy that is the state takes aid into account when devising and implementing policies. Insofar as it is accountable, then, the state must in part be accountable to outside constituencies

(donors). Accountability here means that the state meets the conditions under which aid is delivered. Because dependence (aid) is now so central to the survival and operation of African states, accountability to aid-donors is a priority even if it is at the expense of accountability to domestic constituencies. (p. 243)

Conditionality was particularly strongly enforced during the structural adjustment reforms of the 1980s and 1990s, but more recently, there has been a retreat from direct conditions placed on aid.[1] Yet concerns remain over the ways in which donor influence can undermine state sovereignty, alter political priorities, or impose new power relationships in less explicit, but equally important ways. Swedlund (2013), for instance, evaluates the shift from project based (so-called 'vertical') funding to budgetary support (often termed 'horizontal' funding) in Rwanda and Tanzania to assess if this approach has reduced donor policy influence. He finds that, contrary to popular opinion, donors were also using general budgetary support as a mechanism to shape local policy priorities.

In addition to concerns about influence over policy priorities and choices, some development scholars critique how the international community has fundamentally shaped the *governing institutions* of low-income countries. The historical legacy of colonialism has provided a starting point for some authors to consider how it provided the political, institutional and administrative bases for the construction of the post-colonial state (c.f. Chazan et al. 1999; Mamdani 1997). It is also well known that international financial institutions and donors have played a major role in steering political and institutional development in some countries, explicitly linking the provision of foreign aid with political reform and constitutional change (Stokke 2013). While approaches to international development have changed over the past two decades, with increasing emphasis on the importance of national governance and stewardship, there are still concerns over external influence on governance structures and systems. Harrison (2001) presents the idea of 'post-conditionality' as a situation in which donor-recipient relationships become more subtle than in past conditionality situations (in terms of direct coercion or explicit demands for policy decisions in return for aid). Instead, in systems of post-conditionality, influence is mediated through more informal yet pervasive

---

[1] With some notable exceptions, such as the US government's so-called 'global gag rule' that refuses to provide aid funding to agencies that inform about abortion services in any way, which is repeatedly imposed or rescinded depending on whether a Republican or Democrat is elected as President (Crane and Dusenberry 2004).

practices of administrative guidance, which often embed donor values or ideas into decision structures and reflect power imbalances in doing so. Harrison explains:

> Donors do not just impose conditionalities; they also work in routinized fashion at the centre of policy-making. Donor-funded technical assistance introduces not new policies but new methodologies of policy design based on corporate plans, surveys, and closer budgeting and monitoring techniques. (p. 671)

He further notes that this approach works to establish political relations which make the distinction between external and national level actors less useful as donors become involved within multiple forms and processes of decision making (p. 675). Such insights mirror arguments made by Chambers and Pettit (2004) who have described aid as a 'complex system' in which power relations are reinforced through "[o]rganisational norms and procedures, combined with personal behaviour, attitudes and beliefs (p. 137)."

Within the realm of global health and development, such arrangements can place into potential conflict two sets of institutions – national institutions guided by Ministries of Health, serving local populations, and international global health institutions – each with their own different accountability mechanisms or ultimate goals. Some examples of this have been seen elsewhere. Storeng and Béhague (2014), for instance, identified how particular quantitative indicators were embraced or utilised by international maternal health advocates when these helped increase the global profile of their preferred health issue (so-called 'evidence based advocacy'). Béhague et al. (2009) further have explored how the dominant ideas of what an 'evidence based' policy response should be in maternal and neonatal care could impose global policy interests over domestic ones, pushing countries to generic interventions over tailored implementation strategies and serving to legitimate, rather than inform, key policy stakeholders.

Akin to this, Shiffman (2014) has described the advisory role of key global health actors and networks as an exercise in 'epistemic power' in the ways that it establishes the dominance of particular discourses, priorities and approaches in health policy agendas in low-income settings without necessarily raising questions about the legitimacy or accountability of these actors.

These perspectives thus highlight the salient features of the aid-receiving context in which evidence is both generated and used to guide policy development. We can use these ideas to specifically investigate the institutionalised organisational norms, procedures, behaviours, attitudes and beliefs (to use Chamvers and Pettit's terms) that are established in each setting which shape the utilisation of evidence for health policy decision making.

Evidence Use as a Power/Knowledge Nexus

Despite the existence of a well-established body of both empirical and conceptual work exploring how donors influence structures, processes, and outcomes of policy decision making, these insights are rarely incorporated in debates about, and recommendations to support, the use of evidence in the health sector. Many global actors use an overtly technical language when referring to the use of evidence, at times mirroring ideas of the public health community: presenting evidence as a technical tool that is principally discussed in terms of how it improves the efficiency or effectiveness of programmatic planning and implementation (c.f. WHO 2004; Yamey and Volmink 2014); and donor funds have increasingly been channelled to programmes aiming to 'improve' evidence use principally based on technical arguments (c.f. iDSI undated; UKAid 2014; ODI 2013).

Seeing the role of evidence as simply technical, however, stands in contrast to critical scholars who have explored the decidedly political nature of evidence utilisation (in both public health and other policy realms). Stewart and Smith (2015) for example have recently discussed how particular 'evidence tools' – including systematic reviews, impact assessments or economic decision-support tools (such as cost-effectiveness analyses) – serve political functions in addition to the provision of technical guidance, "primarily in their symbolic value as markers of good decision making"(p. 415). This includes conveying credibility to external audiences as well as providing clear and quantifiable answers to policy questions. Through interviews with public health policy stakeholders, Stewart and Smith found that these tools reflected a high degree of what Weiss (1979) has described as the 'symbolic' use of research – providing signals of what might be considered important, rather than necessarily functioning in the 'problem solving' or 'engineering' roles that many tools are often described as representing.

Ferlie and McGivern (2013) similarly described the field of evidence-based medicine in the UK as a 'power/knowledge nexus' to explore the political implications of promotion of particular ways to utilise evidence to inform health decisions. In a separate paper, Ferlie and colleagues explain:

> power resides in mundane day to day practices, dominant languages, obedient and reformed subjects and taken for granted rationalities. Such power is seen in neutral rather than critical neo Marxist terms: it can constitute a capacity to govern (Clegg, Courpasson, & Phillips, 2006; Townley, 1998) without crude force, domination or exploitation. (Ferlie et al. 2012, p. 340)

In line with the conceptual approach outlined in Chap. 1 of this volume, this chapter explores the application of health policy-relevant knowledge as an exercise of power, pulling out insights from three country cases – Cambodia, Ghana, and Ethiopia – to explore the use of evidence to inform health policy. Our analysis discusses a set of key themes seen in the mechanisms through which donors may influence policy and politics through evidence utilisation, exploring the political and governance implications seen arising from international donors' promotion or utilisation of particular tools and strategies of evidence application to influence health policy.

COMPARATIVE ANALYSIS

The remainder of this chapter attempts to draw out themes about how donor activities or power relationships can have implications for the use of evidence in health policymaking based on our three country investigations undertaken in aid-dependent settings. Each of these countries is also represented in separate chapters of this book, which provide further information and lines of analysis. So, for example, Chap. 2 presents a comparison of evidence use in Cambodia for three different health policy issues: tobacco control, HIV/AIDS, and performance-based financing including the Government Midwifery Incentive Scheme. The chapter finds that the use of evidence for differing policy issues was best explained by mapping out how the various health policy issues differed in terms of the outcomes of concern to key stakeholders; but also by exploring the structurally established positions of influence that stakeholders had, and the logics held by influential stakeholders over which evidence was held to be relevant to any given outcome. Further work arising from our Cambodia research (published elsewhere) looked more broadly at the routes through which donors could have influence over the health policymaking process (analysed through a comparison of Cambodia and Pakistan). That work found that donors could exert influence at each stage of the policy process: priority setting, policy formulation, and policy implementation, monitoring and evaluation. The analysis found that direct funding to preferred policy issues was the most common means of donor influence, but other means of influence arose from control over technical knowledge as well as more indirect influence – such as through financing particular research or evaluations (thus constructing evidence that could be seen as policy relevant), or through recipient country concerns over maintain a good reputation to avoid impacts on non-health areas of concern (e.g. tourism or trade) (Khan et al. 2018).

Influence over institutions and norms by donors can also be seen in the case study from Ghana presented in Chap. 4, which particularly draws out the ways that donors could influence the collection of routine data and indicators to inform annual performance reviews and subsequent sectoral plans. Chapter 3, which presents findings from our Ethiopian case study, looked more specifically at the issue of nutrition policy, and found that the international community's framing of nutrition problems and policy responses could be important factors in helping to explain how evidence was utilised within policymaking processes for that specific issue.

As discussed above, it is important to consider the underlying structural governing dynamics in aid-recipient areas to understand donor influence, including the organisational norms, procedures, or beliefs held that shaping the generation and utilisation of evidence. Through the three case studies in countries reliant on donor support to the health sector, we have thus been able to reflect on multiple ways that donor influence can manifest itself within the structures and processes of evidence use for health policymaking. In this section we draw out three themes that point to particular mechanisms though which donor organisations influence the policy process: through the creation of policy-relevant evidence; through the utilisation of evidence for specific policy processes; and through the construction of systems and routines that shape how evidence informs policy within health policymaking more broadly.

The Generation or Creation of Policy Relevant Evidence

Health sector planning typically requires assessments of the health status and health care needs of a population as well as knowledge about what is feasible or achievable based on different intervention strategies (Abel-Smith

1994; Green 2007). For each of these, however, there may be more or less robust bodies of evidence available to provide information about health care needs and intervention possibilities. As social epidemiologist Nancy Krieger (1992) has stated, "If you don't ask, you don't know, and if you don't know, you can't act (p. 412)." In this way, decisions about which data to collect, the identification of a research agenda and the choice of research topics can be seen to be inherently political as it shapes the topics that enter the agenda, and thus which pathways of policy action can be followed (see also: Parkhurst 2016, 2017).

In Cambodia, it was reported that the research agenda and the availability of routine data from the national health information system are driven by external funding, often focused on high profile diseases (such as malaria or HIV/AIDS), and this could result in the neglect of other important health concerns (with issues like hepatitis, road traffic accidents, or dengue fever mentioned). One interviewee further explained that mental health was another key priority in Cambodia, given the historical legacy of the genocide perpetuated in the 1970s; yet research and policy attention to mental health were said to be lacking due to dependence on donor agendas (see (Khan et al. 2018) for more details). Similarly, a recent literature review found that few research reports on non-communicable diseases in Cambodia have been published, despite these accounting for the highest morbidity and mortality rates in the country (Goyet et al. 2015).

In Ethiopia, the influence of donors was said to arise through their funding to local universities conducting research – through which local evidence would then be generated for health topics of interest to donors (with nutrition given as an example). Paralleling a respondent in Cambodia, an Ethiopian interviewee stated that donor research interests might focus on diseases with a high profile on the global health agenda (such as HIV or TB) without work on lesser known areas which might be important from a national perspective, leading to these topics being overlooked when it comes to the drafting of health policies. Research conducted by development partners or NGOs was also seen to be valued by decision makers more highly than that generated solely by Ethiopian scholars, viewing international partners as experts and potentially excluding local sources of evidence, and thus local voices, from having influence on policymaking.

Cambodian interviewers noted other ways that donors might influence the creation of policy relevant evidence. First, donors were seen as influencing which areas of health information systems were strengthened – thus building capacity to collect and generate routine data for selected areas of health which they prioritised, such as malaria or HIV. Second, donor choice in financing of programme evaluations would again affect which evidence is created in ways that could shape where future policy attention could lie.

Evidence Use Within the Policy Process

A second theme we explore in our case studies focusses on the use of evidence within different health policymaking processes, to consider the roles or influence of donor agencies within these more specific policy decision situations. One of the most well established (yet often critiqued) mechanisms of donor influence in low-income settings is in the direct funding of particular programmes and shaping of national priorities (Buse and Harmer 2007; Ooms et al. 2008; Sridhar and Tamashiro 2009). While there have been shifts away from such so-called vertical programming, it still does occur in many cases, with large numbers of global bodies directing money to specific health issues. Such arrangements can subsequently have direct impacts on evidence use, however, as those issues which received funding for programmatic use could have increased attention to, or application of, particular forms of evidence.

For example, in Cambodia, we investigated three health (system) topics that have recently received policy attention. Of these, it was HIV/AIDS – in comparison to tobacco control or financial performance incentives to health workers – that respondents typically described as having the most robust system to draw on high-quality scientific evidence to guide programmatic decisions; including epidemiological modelling, cost-effectiveness data, and scaling up from pilot programme evaluations. A reason given for this, however, was the interest and support of donors to HIV/AIDS in the country. This included provision of financial and human capacity resources to the bodies planning HIV activities, such as the National Centre for HIV/AIDS, Dermatology and STDs.

It may not be surprising that donor interest in HIV enabled a system of evidence use judged by local actors to be better than in other health decisions. Cambodia has limited human resources for the generation and analysis of policy-relevant evidence. In the other two cases explored in Chap. 2, powerful national interests were seen as dominating the framing of the policy question, which subsequently affected which pieces of evidence were held to be relevant or applied. With the case of tobacco policy, it was industry and national revenue interests that influenced which evidence could be brought to bear; while the Prime Minister's office's direct interest in maternal mortality was seen to shape how a midwifery incentive scheme was conceptualised and how it subsequently used evidence. In the case of HIV/AIDS policy in Cambodia, some saw this as presenting a positive development given the limited or piecemeal application of evidence to inform decisions for other health issues. But there are still challenges in the fact that it might only be a sub-set of issues for which there is a robust enough body of evidence generated, reviewed, or applied to justify international interest and funding.

Furthermore, while it was financing of interventions, and of research on priority topics, that affected evidence use for the agenda-setting stage, donors were also seen to have influence on the policy formulation stage in Cambodia. At this stage, influence was seen to derive from donor proficiency in analysing data and using research outputs to inform policies and plans, or in filling knowledge gaps that might exist – either by commissioning additional research or using their own expertise.

Another example of how international actors may have political influence within specific health policy issues can be seen in Ethiopia. Chapter 3 presents a case study of nutrition planning, exploring how the conceptual framing of nutrition by the global community had implications for how particular evidence could inform policy development. For instance it was explained that international stakeholders and processes, including a 2008 *Lancet* special series on maternal and child undernutrition, led to a common understanding of a need to address nutrition through a multi-sectoral approach. Yet the implications of this were that particular forms of evidence resonated with particular institutionalised logics of appropriateness and were not appropriate for the logics of others, thus hampering efforts to achieve multisectoral policy to address nutrition.

So, for example, it was reported that the Ministry of Agriculture pursued a logic dictated by concern over farm outputs, while the Finance Ministry considered monetary data to justify action from an economic development perspective – in contrast to the typical public health indicators (such as under-five mortality or obesity rates) that are institutionally understood and used to raise malnutrition awareness and priority in global health circles.

The mention of *the Lancet's* 2008 undernutrition series by our interviewees reflects Shiffman's (2014) recent description of epistemic and normative power in global health. Shiffman specifically identifies *the Lancet* as "one of the most powerful actors in global health (p. 298)," in the ways it has worked to set the global agenda and construct ideas of what should be done in health. Our research described in Chap. 3 illustrates this in practice, showing how a special series of that journal worked to shape the conceptual understanding of malnutrition, with subsequent implications for which evidence was drawn upon and how to shape policy development.

Systems and Routines of Evidence Utilisation

As noted in the introduction to this chapter, Harrison's (2001) analysis of 'post-conditionality' identified how donor influence has shifted to routinised processes of policy design. While Harrison focusses on Uganda and Tanzania, he points to a set of other African countries that might fit this description (including Ghana). And from a new institutional perspective (c.f. Lowndes 2010; Peters 2005), routinisation would be reflected in the structures, processes, and norms that shape the use of evidence to inform health policy.

For example, the analysis of Ghana presented in Chap. 4 principally focusses on an institutional process and system for data utilisation to inform health policy and planning – specifically exploring how routine local data and locally relevant research evidence are utilised to populate a set of 'indicators' that are then used to evaluate health sector achievement and inform annual formal sector strategic planning meetings. Using routine data to inform annual planning cycles is of course not an unusual idea, yet it was the specific role of donors in defining indicators, and influencing how they were used to assess national policies, that served as mechanisms by which donors could collectively shape the development of national policy. In particular, it was an annual 'health summit' event during which indicators were developed and populated with data to judge policy success, and steer policy directions for the future.

This example echoes forms of influence described by Whitfield (2007) who explains:

> Donors exhibit powerful influence over policy not only through conditionality, but also through policy dialogue arenas. Donors have created a plethora of arenas for what they call 'policy dialogue' with government, as well as for coordinating their operations, sharing information and experience, discussing policies, and identifying opportunities to engage government on policy reforms. (p. 145)

Such policy dialogues can be particularly fertile environments for the introduction of 'evidence' when conceptualised in a technical problem solving manner, with the form, location, and arrangements around such dialogues having implications for power and influence within the local settings.

In Cambodia, however, there were also examples of structured processes and routinised norms that reflected donor influence on the broader institutional environment that shaped evidence use within health policymaking for any number of policy decisions. In Cambodia, for instance, one respondent explained that technical reports were typically published in English, creating an immediate barrier for some local stakeholders to engage with technical evidence. It was also reported that research was driven by funding rather than local demand, which could mean available research could be less relevant to the country. This shows some similarity to issues raised in Ethiopia where it was reported that internationally produced evidence is more respected than that produced internally by national institutions.

Discussion: Influence and Resistance Over Multiple Forms of Evidence Use

The influence of donors in aid-recipient nations has long been a subject of interest to development scholars, yet rarely have these issues directly been analysed in relation to issues of evidence use within the policy process. Our comparative analysis identified a range of examples and themes through which donor influence could manifest itself in shaping the way evidence was generated or utilised to inform decisions, as well as in the ongoing systems or routines that can influence evidence use as well.

As noted in Chap. 1, Carol Weiss described multiple meanings of research utilisation in the 1970s (c.f. Weiss 1979) – including rational 'problem solving' uses of research, but also how research serves a 'knowledge driven' role to identify problems in the first place, or to influence broader thinking about issues through a so-called 'enlightenment' mechanism. The case studies explored in this chapter illustrate examples of evidence and research use fitting each of these meanings. Influence over evidence generation, for example, could shape the knowledge construction process which serves to identify health problems for policy attention in the first place. The direct support to priority issues, on the other hand, allowed certain topics to have evidence used more robustly in a classic problem solving modality. Influence over broader systems of data use, or routinised norms related to expertise and evidence utilisation, on the other hand, might alternatively reflect Weiss' enlightenment ideas.

In these ways we can of course consider donor influence as an exercise of power. The historical concern of some authors over donor control of resources (i.e. funding) certainly was found to be a major influence on which issues received attention, which at times shaped which health issues were seen to have had robust or improved evidence utilisation processes as well. Yet power also could be seen as present in the expert knowledge and capacity in regards to evidence utilisation that international actors possessed, or were perceived as possessing – so called epistemic power linked to scientific expertise.

This said, our country cases also illustrated a number of ways that donor power and influence might be resisted – themes particularly discussed in Ghana and Ethiopia. At the time of the research, Ghana was the only one of our three aid-dependent settings classified as a lower-middle income country (today Cambodia also falls into this classification), but Ghana particularly stood out as having greater local capacity related to evidence generation and use than in Ethiopia or Cambodia. Multiple respondents in Ghana referred to significant research or evidence generative capacity in national bodies, including the Ghana Health Service (GHS) as well as universities. One interviewee stated that the country had a strong desire to be independent from donors in its desire to rely on local data for evaluations; and in another case a representative of a UN body stated that they choose research topics based on those requested by the government.

Notably, there are three well-regarded Health Research Centres within the Research and Development Division of the GHS, serving the northern, middle, and southern regions of the country. According to national documents, these centres conduct research within their designated subregion as per the needs and priorities of the GHS, this information is then used to guide national-level decision making and policy development (Ghana Health Service 2015). All centres are also said to have well established health and demographic surveillance systems and collaborate with a number of international partners and funders (Ghana Health Service 2015; Navrongo Health Research Centre 2016). In contrast, in Cambodia and Ethiopia, there were indications that donors had a strong say over which health topics were researched in the first place. Thus the generation of policy-relevant data could be seen to follow donor interests with subsequent implications for policy options. Ghana, however, with its higher capacity and better established research and bureaucratic bodies, appeared less susceptible to influence in this way.

Despite greater local capacity in Ghana, interviewees still mentioned donors could shape policy decisions – achieved through their allocation of resources to specific issues, through a national desire to appease donors so as to maintain budgets, or even through lobbying for preferred policies. One representative of the GHS interviewed noted that there still will be priority allocated to issues based on the power of stakeholders – providing an example of how breast cancer was addressed before cervical cancer in the country, as it affects wealthier individuals, despite representing a lower burden of disease in the country. Yet Ghana has been noted elsewhere for having established a muti-donor budget support mechanism and associated policy dialogue mechanism to improve coordination of aid and maintain national leadership of policymaking in the face of donor proliferation (Pallas et al. 2015). As such there appeared to be a tension between the capacity and strength of local decision making systems and the influence of donors at multiple points.

In Ethiopia, as noted, local capacity was acknowledged as weak for much health planning and decision making. Yet despite the fact that we identified influence over evidence creation and framing of issue responses by donors and international actors, Ethiopian policymaking and planning was understood to be strongly centrally controlled, which seemed to indicate significant resistance to direct influence over decisions or priority setting at times. Indeed, in a recent assessment of potential donor influence on policy in Ethiopia over two decades, Borchgrevink (2008) found particularly strong resistance to influence in the country. A key explanation the author gives is how:

> the Ethiopian regime is independent-minded, proud, and unwilling to bow to the whims and wishes of donors and the international community in general. The [ruling coalition] has learnt self-reliance during a long guerrilla struggle, has a strong commitment to its own development model with a basis in Marxism-Leninism, and a perhaps healthy distrust of the reliability of donors. (p. 216)

This, in combination with a lack of donor coordination or consistency and the lack of significant threat to change the regime, are used by Borchgrevink to explain that "donors have been relatively powerless to influence Ethiopian policies (p. 215)." Indeed, one representative of a UN agency stated that it was still the Ethiopian government who decides how to use the results of research programmes, for instance, even if research was supported externally. This difficulty to influence the government was also reflected in several of our interviews, where the strength of the government was seen to limit the influence donors could have – both on policy agendas, but also on the roles that evidence plays in planning.

Ultimately, insights from multiple countries illustrate balances between donor influence and national country resistance or control over policymaking. Agendas could be directly shaped by donor funds, or more indirectly influenced through creation of policy-relevant evidence. Yet the extent and impact of each of these was contextually determined, influenced by government capacity, systems, and control over aspects of decision making in the health sector. Strategic forms of resistance to influence would also reflect the idea of aid as a 'game' situation, explored in earlier work on aid conditionality by Mosely et al. (1995) in which donors and recipients are conceptualised as pursuing different goals, basing behaviour on the expected response of the other party and potential trade-offs as a result.

CONCLUSIONS

While the use of evidence to inform health policy has often been discussed in technical terms, critical policy scholars have noted how such conceptualisations may mask or ignore important aspects of policymaking – including how evidence promotion or utilisation risks depoliticising the policy process – both by obscuring the fundamental value-based choices that policy makers must consider and trade off, as well as obscuring the governance implications that may arise from the different ways evidence may be used to steer or shape ultimate policy decisions. Exploring these concerns through the specific context of aid-dependent settings, however, adds new insights into how power dynamics can play out in multiple ways affecting not only specific policy decision making, but also through the underlying governing institutional structures that shape how evidence is created, selected, or interpreted to inform policy decisions.

In our comparative reflection presented above, the political-economy of aid and development has been shown to manifest itself through a number of more or less visible processes of evidence utilisation. Donor agencies not only use evidence to essentially promote desired policy choices and agenda topics, but they similarly have influence over which policy-relevant evidence bases are created in the first place by funding research, strengthening select routine data sources, or undertaking programmatic evaluations of desired interventions. They further have been shown to have influence over the ways that pieces of evidence are interpreted in decision making fora at times, illustrating the power dynamics within decisions around which evidence is relevant for what policy and planning considerations. Finally, donors at times work to construct institutionalised systems and processes, the continuing performance of which may work to prioritise particular problems, solutions, or power relationships within the health sector. In all these ways we can see the importance of critically investigating the power and governance implications of evidence promotion and use, particularly in low and middle income settings which have historically had less research in these areas, yet which clearly show important dynamics as well due to the political dynamics of the aid donor-recipient relationship.

REFERENCES

Abel-Smith, Brian. 1994. *An introduction to health: Policy, planning and financing*. London: Longman.

Behague, Dominique, Charlotte Tawiah, Mikey Rosato, Telesphore Some, and Joanna Morrison. 2009. Evidence-based policy-making: The implications of globally-applicable research for context-specific problem-solving in developing countries. *Social Science & Medicine* 69 (10): 1539–1546.

Borchgrevink, Axel. 2008. Limits to donor influence: Ethiopia, aid and conditionality. *Forum for Development Studies* 35 (2): 195–220. https://doi.org/10.10 80/08039410.2008.9666409.

Buse, Kent, and Andrew M. Harmer. 2007. Seven habits of highly effective global public–private health partnerships: Practice and potential. *Social Science & Medicine* 64 (2): 259–271.

Chabal, Patrick. 1992. *Power in Africa*. London: Macmillian Press Ltd.

Chambers, Robert, and Jethro Pettit. 2004. Shifting power to make a difference. In *Inclusive aid: Changing power and relationships in international development*, ed. Leslie Groves and Rachel Hinton, 137–162. London: Earthscan.

Chazan, Naomi, Peter Lewis, Robert Mortimer, Donald Rothchild, and Stephen John Stedman. 1999. *Politics and society in contemporary Africa*. 3rd ed. Boulder: Lynne Rienner Publishers, Inc.

Crane, Barbara B., and Jennifer Dusenberry. 2004. Power and politics in international funding for reproductive health: The US global gag rule. *Reproductive Health Matters* 12 (24): 128–137. https://doi.org/10.1016/S0968-8080(04)24140-4.

Ferlie, Ewan, and Gerry McGivern. 2013. Bringing Anglo-governmentality into public management scholarship: The case of evidence-based medicine in UK health care. *Journal of Public Administration Research and Theory.* https://doi.org/10.1093/jopart/mut002.
Ferlie, Ewan, Gerry Mcgivern, and Louise FitzGerald. 2012. A new mode of organizing in health care? Governmentality and managed networks in cancer services in England. *Social Science & Medicine* 74 (3): 340–347.
Ghana Health Service. 2015. Research and development division: Research centres. http://www.ghanahealthservice.org/division-scat.php?ghsdid=11&ghsscid=68. Accessed 28 Nov 2016.
Goyet, Sophie, Socheat Touch, Por Ir, Sovannchhorvin SamAn, Thomas Fassier, Roger Frutos, Arnaud Tarantola, and Hubert Barennes. 2015. Gaps between research and public health priorities in low income countries: Evidence from a systematic literature review focused on Cambodia. *Implementation Science* 10 (1): 32.
Green, Andrew. 2007. *An introduction to health planning for developing health systems.* Oxford: Oxford University Press.
Harrison, Graham. 2001. Post-conditionality politics and administrative reform: Reflections on the cases of Uganda and Tanzania. *Development and Change* 32 (4): 657–679.
iDSI. undated. About us. NICE-International. http://www.idsihealth.org/about-us/. Accessed 8 June 2015.
Khan, Mishal S., Ankita Meghani, Marco Liverani, Imara Roychowdhury, and Justin Parkhurst. 2018. Influences of external donors on national health policy processes: Experiences of local policy actors in Cambodia and Pakistan. *Health Policy and Planning.* 33 (2): 215–223. https://doi.org/10.1093/heapol/czx145
Koeberle, Stefan G. 2003. Should policy-based lending still involve conditionality? *The World Bank Research Observer* 18 (2): 249–273. https://doi.org/10.1093/wbro/lkg009.
Krieger, Nancy. 1992. The making of public health data: Paradigms, politics, and policy. *Journal of Public Health Policy* 13: 412–427.
Lancaster, Carol. 2008. *Foreign aid: Diplomacy, development, domestic politics.* Chicago: University of Chicago Press.
Lowndes, Vivian. 2010. The institutional approach. In *Theory and methods in political science,* ed. David Marsh and Gerry Stoker, 6–79. Basingstoke: Palgrave Macmillian.
Mamdani, Mahmood. 1997. *Citizen and subject: Decentralised despotism and the legacy of late colonialism.* Delhi: Oxford University Press.
McDougall, Derek. 2011. Australia's engagement with its 'near abroad': A change of direction under the Labor government, 2007–10? *Commonwealth & Comparative Politics* 49 (3): 318–341. https://doi.org/10.1080/14662043.2011.582735.

Mosley, Paul, Jane Harringan, and John Toye. 1995. *Aid and power: Second edition: The World Bank & policy-based lending*. Vol. 1. London: Routledge.
Navrongo Health Research Centre. 2016. Partners & funders. http://www.navrongo-hrc.org/content/partners-funders. Accessed 28 Nov 2016.
ODI. 2013. Australia-Indonesia partnership for pro-poor policy: The knowledge sector initiative. Overseas Development Institute. http://www.odi.org/projects/2677-australia-indonesia-partnership-pro-poor-policy-knowledge-sector-initiative. Accessed 8 June 2015.
Okuonzi, Sam Agatre, and Joanna Macrae. 1995. Whose policy is it anyway? International and national influences on health policy development in Uganda. *Health Policy and Planning* 10 (2): 122–132.
Ooms, Gorik, Wim Van Damme, Brook K. Baker, Paul Zeitz, and Ted Schrecker. 2008. The 'diagonal' approach to Global Fund financing: A cure for the broader malaise of health systems? *Globalization and Health* 4 (6): 1–7.
Pallas, Sarah Wood, Justice Nonvignon, Moses Aikins, and Jennifer Prah. 2015. Responses to donor proliferation in Ghana's health sector: A qualitative case study. *Bulletin of the World Health Organization* 93: 11–18.
Parkhurst, Justin. 2017. *The politics of evidence: from evidence based policy to the good governance of evidence*. Abingdon: Routledge.
Parkhurst, Justin O. 2016. Appeals to evidence for the resolution of wicked problems: The origins and mechanisms of evidentiary bias. *Policy Sciences* 49 (4): 373–393. https://doi.org/10.1007/s11077-016-9263-z.
Peters, Guy. 2005. *Institutional theory in political science*. London: Continuum.
Shiffman, Jeremy. 2014. Knowledge, moral claims and the exercise of power in global health. *International Journal of Health Policy and Management* 3 (6): 297–299. https://doi.org/10.15171/ijhpm.2014.120.
Sridhar, Devi, and Tami Tamashiro. 2009. Vertical funds in the health sector: Lessons for education from the Global Fund and GAVI. United Nations Educational, Scientific and Cultural Organization (UNESCO).
Stewart, Ellen, and Katherine E. Smith. 2015. 'Black magic' and 'gold dust': The epistemic and political uses of evidence tools in public health policy making. *Evidence & Policy: A Journal of Research, Debate and Practice* 11 (3): 415–437. https://doi.org/10.1332/174426415X14381786400158.
Stokke, Olav. 2013. *Aid and political conditionality*. London: Frank Cass & Co. Ltd.
Storeng, Katerini T., and Dominique P. Béhague. 2014. "Playing the numbers game": Evidence-based advocacy and the technocratic narrowing of the safe motherhood initiative. *Medical Anthropology Quarterly* 28 (2): 260–279.
Swedlund, Haley J. 2013. From donorship to ownership? Budget support and donor influence in Rwanda and Tanzania. *Public Administration and Development* 33 (5): 357–370.
UKAid. 2014. BCURE building capacity to use research evidenve. http://wordpress.com/. Accessed 2 Oct 2014.

Van Belle, Douglas A. 2004. *Media, bureaucracies, and foreign aid: A comparative analysis of the United States, the United Kingdom, Canada, France and Japan.* New York: Palgrave Macmillan.

Weiss, Carol H. 1979. The many meanings of research utilization. *Public Administration Review* 39 (5): 426–431.

Whitfield, Lindsay. 2007. Identity construction in development practices: The government of Ghana, civil society, private sector, and development partners. In *Professional identities: Policy and practice at work in business and bureaucracy*, ed. Shirley Ardener and Fiona Moore, 143–160. New York: Berghahn Books.

WHO. 2004. *World report on knowledge for better health: Strengthening health systems.* Geneva: World Health Organization.

World Bank. Net ODA received (% of GNI). https://data.worldbank.org/indicator/DT.ODA.ODAT.GN.ZS. Accessed 12 Jan 2017.

Yamey, Gavin, and Jimmy Volmink. 2014. An argument for evidence-based policymaking in global health. In *The handbook of global health policy*, ed. Garett W. Brown, Gavin Yamey, and Sarah Wamala, 133–155. Chichester: Wiley-Blackwell.

Open Access This chapter is licensed under the terms of the Creative Commons Attribution 4.0 International License (http://creativecommons.org/licenses/by/4.0/), which permits use, sharing, adaptation, distribution and reproduction in any medium or format, as long as you give appropriate credit to the original author(s) and the source, provide a link to the Creative Commons license and indicate if changes were made.

The images or other third party material in this chapter are included in the chapter's Creative Commons license, unless indicated otherwise in a credit line to the material. If material is not included in the chapter's Creative Commons license and your intended use is not permitted by statutory regulation or exceeds the permitted use, you will need to obtain permission directly from the copyright holder.

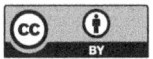

CHAPTER 11

Conclusion: Reflecting on Studying Evidence Use from a Public Policy Perspective

Justin Parkhurst, Benjamin Hawkins, and Stefanie Ettelt

Returning to the Question: What Does It Mean to Use Evidence in Policymaking?

As Chap. 1 of this volume noted, the growth in interest in the use of evidence in policymaking has been remarkable in recent years. Nowhere has this been truer than in the area of health policy, given the close affiliation and historical associations with the evidence based medicine movement. There has been a proliferation of formal structures, bodies, processes and mechanisms within government and policy making designed to facilitate the use of evidence in decision making. Examples include new government agencies mandated with evidence synthesis, the establishment of health technology appraisal bodies, or the creation of standalone bodies at arm's length or independent from government, providing syntheses for

---

J. Parkhurst (✉)
London School of Economics and Political Science, London, UK
e-mail: j.parkhurst@lse.ac.uk

B. Hawkins • S. Ettelt
London School of Hygiene and Tropical Medicine, London, UK
e-mail: ben.hawkins@lshtm.ac.uk; stefanie.ettelt@lshtm.ac.uk

public policy information (such as the UK's 'what works centres'). Reflecting these developments, there has been a commensurate expansion in focus on the idea and practice of evidence use in policymaking amongst both scholars and practitioners. This is evident in the emergence, and increasing profile, of journals focussed specifically on evidence utilisation, such as *Evidence & Policy* or *Implementation Science*, and international events such as the *Global Evidence Summit* or the *What Works Global Summit* which are now held on a regular basis. The desire to engage with questions surrounding evidence use appears greater than ever.

Despite these important developments, the field of work looking at evidence use in policymaking appears to still be in its infancy, with scholars struggling to make sense of evidence use in real world settings. Policy scholars studying efforts made to achieve 'uptake' of research findings are often struck by the use of the language of 'evidence-based policy' in both academic and professional circles with little, if any, explicit definition of what counts as 'evidence' and what it means to have that evidence 'taken up' in policy decisions. At times, it seems easier to identify a policy community advocating for 'evidence-based policymaking', than to find clarity on what the term actually means. As discussed elsewhere (Parkhurst 2017), many champions of 'evidence based policy making' express explicit concern with problematic ways that evidence is used. This includes criticisms that policy makers ignore relevant evidence in decision making, or engage in 'cherry-picking' or manipulation of evidence for strategic ends. Yet the identification of unscientific practices and problems of bias in some political processes does not produce conceptual clarity about what real world practices of evidence use in policy making look like and, from a normative perspective, what they *should* look like.

Improving conceptual clarity requires a more nuanced understanding of the process of evidence production, the epistemological status of research outputs (i.e. the types of knowledge claims which are substantiated by a given study or piece of evidence) and the process of evidence use. Reflecting this, many policy scholars interested in questions of evidence use have shifted from a discourse of 'evidence based' to 'evidence informed' policymaking reflecting the realisation that evidence is one influence on policy amongst many (including ideological orientation of governments and societies and the political priorities and consent over the direction of policy by the populations affected by decisions). Moreover, the shift in language reflects the realisation that, while evidence can guide decisions, or inform us about the likely consequences of policy choices, it cannot guide what policy objectives governments *ought* to choose. This is particularly the case where governments face often mutually exclusive choices between competing policy agendas promoted by multiple policy advocates in the contexts of finite resources.

Chapter 1 also noted that there have been many attempts to identify the multiple ways research or evidence might influence policy, with works by those such as Carol Weiss (1979, 1982, 1991), or Sandra Nutley, Huw Davies and colleagues (see Davies et al. 2000; Nutley et al. 2007, 2013) mapping out many of the most common ways that pieces of research or evidence appear to influence decisions. There is also no shortage of systematic reviews that have been conducted attempting to draw together empirical work on the subject, identifying barriers and facilitators to evidence use of one kind or another (c.f. Oliver et al. 2014; Mitton et al. 2007; Contandriopoulos et al. 2010; McCormack et al. 2013). However, there is still a gap in the literature relating to understanding the politics of evidence use, which warrants specific attention to be given to policy processes, the actors involved, the forms of contestation associated with policymaking, and the institutions that shape these processes and, by extension, evidence use.

A public policy perspective can integrate and move beyond initial typologies to understand the ways in which contextual factors shape evidence use in different policy environments. In particular, forms of political contestation around policy problems and their putative solutions, and institutional structures – including political systems in which policy responses are formulated and decisions are taken – shape the use of evidence in health policymaking. In the following sections, we reflect on how the case studies presented in the current volume provide insights into these three areas and into understanding the processes of evidence informed policy making more generally. We conclude with a broader discussion about the possible trajectories of future research agendas on evidence use in policymaking.

INSTRUMENTAL USES OF EVIDENCE

As has been identified previously (Smith 2013a; Russell et al. 2008; Cairney 2016), the public health community's language and thinking about evidence use often reflects Weiss' mostly instrumental meanings of research utilisation (i.e. her 'knowledge-driven' or 'problem-solving' models (Weiss 1979)). Yet politics and political systems tend to result in policy processes that rarely resemble this rational-linear, instrumental model (c.f. Weiss 1979, 1991; Russell et al. 2008; Hammersley 2013).

Our case studies illustrate that there can be particular institutional arrangements in place which make instrumental uses of evidence more likely; arrangements that are typically created for exactly this purpose. The concept of evidence advisory systems, explored in Chap. 8 in particular, points to ways that formalised infrastructures might be deployed to ensure that both a supply of policy relevant evidence is available (e.g. research being undertaken, data collected, or bodies of evidence summarised), and that there are mechanisms through which decision makers can use policy-relevant evidence to inform decision making. We saw such systems have important effects in high income countries, with the Federal Joint Committee (GBA) in Germany and Public Health England being specifically mandated to review the evidence on policies within their remit.

Yet we also saw structural arrangements in lower and middle income settings playing important roles in driving instrumental uses of evidence. In Colombia (see Chap. 5), the implementation of organisations such as IETS (modelled on the example of the English National Institute for Health and Care Excellence (NICE), and tasked with providing health technology assessments similar to NICE) demonstrates the wider applicability of this model and the potential for trans-national knowledge transfer of evidence advisory systems, often via key individuals promoting a particular approach. In Ghana (Chap. 4), we further saw how the established national systems of data collection in healthcare fed into regular annual meetings that used such data to inform the evaluations of the health sector and plan for the future. Yet the Ghanaian case also illustrates that these systems do not remove political considerations or contestation from the processes of evidence use. Indeed, that chapter shows that they can routinise structures with decidedly political implications; with that chapter exploring how donor influence within this system could be seen to challenge local accountability processes. In a similar vein, contestation of evidence in case studies from Germany and England demonstrate that structures built to improve or rationalise evidence use cannot entirely prevent research evidence becoming embroiled in political debate and/or being used strategically to strengthen one side of a debate. Ultimately, we would argue that instrumental use relies on people actively prioritising this type of evidence use, sharing a belief that drawing on findings from research improves the quality of the outcome of decisions. In this sense, institutional structures to support the use of research in policy can work to embed this belief and reflect a willingness to enhance, and invest in, an instrumental role for research in supporting policy decisions.

Political Contestation and Strategic Uses of Evidence

The existence of political contestation around the identification of policy problems and decisions on their proposed solutions, even within formalised advisory systems, underlines the fundamentally political nature of the policy process and the impossibility of stepping outside of politics even in the context of highly technical forms of decision making. Decisions about issues such as the prioritisation of different policy problems in the context of limited resources, or the way to address complex, multi-dimensional health issues which derive from multiple causal factors including those which are hard to define, isolate, and measure (e.g. the social determinants of health), will draw on multiple bodies of evidence – often in different forms and adhering to different epistemological norms. Unavoidably, the decision making process confronts different values, norms and political ideologies, in addition to whatever evidence has been chosen in support of the decision. An example of this is illustrated in the case study in Ethiopia (Chap. 3), whereby the multi-sectoral planning required to address nutrition in that country meant that multiple interests were relevant to a decision, and there were differing views on which evidence was therefore relevant or how to use it to inform decisions.

Yet we have also examined cases illustrating active disagreement between policy stakeholders about policy goals. This contestation could appear visibly, or it could be less explicit. In our aid-recipient nations, for instance, often the conflicts between the aims of international funding bodies and the agendas of national governments were not necessarily publicly debated. Interviews provided insights into how donor funding for particular research topics, or support for the construction of particular pieces of research (such as programmatic evaluations), could shape the evidence base to set policy priorities. Similarly, the political dynamics through which evidence of certain topics was brought to political decision processes was seen in some places as a mechanism for donor influence; as was the influence that could result when donors shaped the processes through which evidence and data are brought to bear on policy decisions (see discussion in Chap. 10; also Khan et al. 2017).

We found overt and explicit contestation more visible in our middle and higher income settings (although the extent to which conflict plays out 'behind the scene' was not investigated per se). In Colombia (Chap. 5), for instance, debates around national health system reform demonstrated the importance of different ideas about the relationship between the individual and the state and the role of the state and private enterprises in funding and providing healthcare in the incremental process of reforming the country's health system. Whilst evidence was called upon by all sides to support their positions, and was cited in draft legislation in support of proposals, it was unable to resolve conflicts between policy actors with deeply entrenched ideological positions.

In England (Chap. 7), we also saw how tobacco control debates around new nicotine delivery systems (e-cigarettes) have polarised the public health community and the strategic use of evidence to support the promotion of very different framing of the policy problem facing government and the regulatory approach it should take in addressing this. Evidence is cited by policy actors and researchers on both sides of the debate. For example, those who see the harm reduction potential of e-cigarettes point to studies showing reduced levels of toxicity in e-cigarette vapour versus tobacco smoke, whilst those taking a tobacco control perspective highlight the lack of epidemiological studies on their long term health effects. At this stage of the debate, with the need for significant additional research needed to remove uncertainty about the long-term health effects of e-cigarettes, recourse to evidence is unable to resolve conflicts between actors who view the issue in fundamentally different terms and from different professional perspectives.

The competitive nature of many policy environments can be seen to drive Weiss' (1979) idea of 'strategic' uses of evidence. In such cases, evidence is seen to be used as 'ammunition' to achieve pre-defined positions or policy goals – fundamentally to 'win' in the competitive process. Using evidence strategically may risk violating established principles of good scientific practice, however. It is also not compatible with notions of 'instrumental' use, although this distinction can be difficult to uphold and might well be part of the contestation. For example, in England, the public health community for many years collaborated effectively to influence government policy on tobacco control, strategically utilising scientific evidence to support their position. This was widely seen to be a legitimate use of evidence. Yet the tobacco industry also routinely engaged in strategic uses of evidence to support arguments in opposition to tobacco control measures, typically in ways judged to be biased by researchers and tobacco control advocates (c.f. Bero 2005; Lee et al. 2004; Ulucanlar et al. 2014).

Even rules-based health governance systems such as Germany's are open to strategic evidence use under conditions of contestation. The case study on minimum volume regulation (Chap. 6) demonstrated that while the Federal Joint Committee, the body mandated with setting minimum volumes, is required by law to appreciate the evidence in support of minimum volumes, its constituting member organisations were pitted against each other, with the German Hospital Association being strongly opposed to such regulation and marshalling its own evidence in support of its position. Evidence in this example was therefore used both instrumentally and strategically.

In our case studies, we found no indication that parliaments (explored in Chap. 9) were particularly prone to use evidence to inform decision (i.e. law) making. While this subject requires substantial additional research, this observation seems to suggest that in settings in which contestation is acted out openly and purposefully, the case for using evidence in an 'objective' or systematic way is harder to make. While there are structures in place in some countries to provide scientific advice to parliamentarians and committees, the emphasis of parliamentary process is on creating majorities and these majorities are typically formed within the context of party politics (although these can play out very differently in different parliamentary cultures as we have seen cross our case studies). There is a debate to be had about the extent to which parliaments should be better informed by evidence. It is certainly desirable for politicians to be literate in research use and for political parties to have their proposals questioned by recourse to evidence. Yet expecting parliament to operate in an 'evidence based' fashion seems to suggest an expectation that it is possible to reduce contestation in (i.e. depoliticise) political debate which is a contradiction in terms. In fact, this is more likely to happen in political systems that intentionally stifle or suppress contestation than in those with established democratic traditions.

The Construction of Issues and Impact on Evidence Use

While there may be both subtle and overt forms of contestation around evidence-informed policy debates, the case studies contained in this volume also point to a larger overarching theme important in shaping the use of evidence in health policy making. In particular, a number of cases explored the fundamental importance of issue construction and issue framing within local contexts in determining when and how evidence is used in the policy process.

It might be expected that certain features of health problems make issues more or less conducive to particular types of evidence use. Such thinking is evident in the health policy literature, with the concept of 'issue characteristics' used by some to help explain global health policy agenda setting or the success of global health networks (Shiffman 2007; Shiffman et al. 2015). The importance of issue characteristics has also been proposed in other policy areas, for example, to understand what is considered rational policymaking in areas like global warming (Oshitani 2013), or to explain different bargaining strategies adopted within the EU by member states (McKibben 2010).

Within the health sector, scholars have argued that certain characteristics of policy issues might influence the ways in which evidence is used in decision making. For example, there is general recognition of cases where issues directly impact on private sector financial interests, which has led to strategic uses of evidence by corporate actors. Examples of this have been widely documented for the tobacco and alcohol industry for instance (Marmot 2004; Smith 2013b; Tong and Glantz 2007; McCambridge et al. 2014). We also see cases where policies are contested in terms of moral arguments about the appropriateness of certain behaviours, including sexual activity and drug use and the appropriate forms of treatment and the extent of resources which should be directed to tackling these conditions. A clear example of this surrounds arguments in favour of and against harm reduction approaches to injecting drug users (c.f Keane 2003; Rhodes et al. 2010; Buchanan et al. 2003), or debates about sexual health (c.f. Epstein 2006; Lyons 1999; Wald et al. 2001).

However, the concept of 'issue characteristics' deployed in much of the health policy literature is problematic, as it can assume an overly materialist and objectivist conception of the nature of social problems and underplays the extent to which policy problems are a result of inter-discursive processes of problem construction by policy actors. Moreover, it is possible that there will be multiple (sometimes starkly conflicting) accounts of the 'same' policy issue within the same policy space. Similarly, we can find examples where seemingly technical issues, for which one might not expect contestation to arise around evidence use, could become problematized in unique ways, resulting in debates over evidence that might not be expected based on the nature of the policy decision (c.f. D'Souza and Parkhurst 2018).

Rather than health issues having inherent characteristics, it is, therefore, more appropriate to explore how different health issues are framed or constructed in particular ways in different settings, and to seek to understand the consequences of this for evidence use. In some of our lower-income fieldwork countries we asked interviewees about whether particular issues were highly contested, including asking about sexual health or HIV specifically. However, we did not find any respondents identifying any strong contestation over these in relation to their (current) work. In a similar vein, our interviews in Ghana identified little contestation or challenge around evidence use and policy formulation for tobacco control in that country – potentially explained by the fact that the country is not a tobacco producer and has relatively low smoking rates. This serves as a reminder that just because an issue may be deeply polarised and highly contested in one setting, it does not mean that the issue is inherently polarising. Nor does it meant that evidence around the issue will be necessarily used strategically, as has been seen with both HIV and tobacco control elsewhere (c.f. Parkhurst 2013; Parkhurst et al. 2015; Smith 2013b; and in Chap. 7 in this volume).

In Cambodia (Chap. 2), policy debates around HIV/AIDS was not found to be characterised by strong contestation along moral lines (according to our interviewees working primarily in national public health roles). Rather, it was presented as an example where evidence was used well in the country by respondents. In this case, 'good evidence use' was seen to be reflected in how international donor communities reviewed and relied on epidemiological studies to guide the choice of interventions for HIV/AIDS locally – a use of evidence that more reflects Weiss' instrumental modes.

Chapter 2 also illustrates just how fluid or dynamic the understanding of the concept of a 'good use' of evidence can be, and how this itself might be a construct of the specific context and policy needs. A second example mentioned by interviewees as exemplifying a good use of evidence was around a national programme providing financial incentives for health workers to encourage pregnant women to deliver in health facilities. When pressed further to explain why this was an exemplar, interviewees explained that there was 'evidence' of a problem of high maternal mortality, and a need to achieve progress towards the millennium development goal of reducing maternal mortality, and this intervention was clearly well targeted to achieve those goals. This conceptualisation of good evidence use for policy, however, is quite different from most conceptualisations in the global public health community. Instead, this judgement appears to have arisen from a broader idea that evidence can identify problems, and a proactive policy response to those problems (regardless of the efficacy of the intervention) would thus provide a good example of evidence use.

Ultimately, our cases, and the broader literature on which they build, point to the ways in which evidence use in policymaking reflect the interaction between processes of issue framing and contestation. Thus, ideas about the appropriate or 'good' use of evidence use are not fixed or universal but vary between policy contexts and even between issues within the same context depending on the way in which a policy problem and their solutions are constructed and the institutional context in which policy decisions are taken.

ADDING INSTITUTIONAL ANALYSIS

From the policy perspective adopted in this volume, political institutions are of central importance to help understand the use of research evidence in health policymaking. Chapter 1 noted that there was a sizable gap in the literature of work exploring the institutional arrangements that work to shape which evidence is used, when, by whom, and to what ends. The chapters in this volume draw out a number of ways that institutions play key roles in shaping policy processes and by extension evidence use for health policymaking, providing a second key area of insight in addition to the nature of political contestation and issue construction.

One way institutions can influence evidence utilisation is by shaping which policy actors are involved in the policy process, or have access to those directly involved, and thus whose positions are considered. This was clearly illustrated in the analysis of Ghana (Chap. 4), where the formal processes of data analysis for policy review routinised the important roles that international donors had in the policy process. The comparative evaluation of evidence advisory systems in Chap. 8 similarly illustrated cases where some key stakeholders might be structured into policy-relevant positions due to institutional arrangements. In Germany's corporatist health governance system, non-state actors such as hospital or sickness fund associations, influence policy directly as they are legally mandated to be part of the top decision-making committee, while other actors have a minor or no role in decision making (e.g. patient organisations are consulted but do not have voting rights). Finally, the comparative analysis presented in Chap. 9 explored how formal authority over particular health decisions could lie with legislatures or judiciaries in countries, with important implications for how evidence would be considered and used as a result. Questions arise as to how these bodies are equipped when dealing with scientific evidence and whether there are limits to what can be achieved in terms of faithfulness to the scientific production of such evidence (Jasanoff and Nelkin 1981).

However, there can be less formal norms and practices that are institutionalised within key policymaking structures which could have implications for evidence use. March and Olsen's (2006) concept of institutional 'logics of appropriateness' can be seen to capture the ways that expectations about evidence, and understandings around how policy-relevant evidence can be embedded within different decision making bodies. Chapter 3 drew explicitly on this concept in Ethiopia to explore how the expectations and norms of evidence use could differ between government sectors, with potential implications for how evidence may or may not be used to inform multi-sectoral planning on nutrition. Similarly, the judicialisation of certain health policy decisions in Colombia (Chap. 5), particularly in relation to the provision of medicines and treatments led to different conceptualisations around what evidence is relevant to inform decisions than was the case in policy deliberations within the legislative-executive nexus (for a more detailed account, see Hawkins and Alvarez Rosete 2017). In Germany, courts grappled with the concept of 'hierarchies of evidence' demanding randomised controlled trials to provide the evidence in support of certain minimum volumes, irrespective of the fact that these studies do not exist and are not feasible to be conducted, especially not in the context of German hospital care. In addition, judicial decisions are typically based on the correct application of legally and constitutionally enshrined rights to specific individuals, but courts may be ill equipped to take account of the wider social and economic consequences of the decision, such as the implications of the ruling in question for resource allocation elsewhere in the system or the overall financial sustainability of the health system (although there are significant differences in legal practice in this respect between countries).

Institutions thus influence the use of evidence in policymaking for health in multiple ways. First, institutional arrangements can provide direction to both thinking and action involving evidence use. For example, the logics of appropriateness embedded within government institutions around evidence may make it more likely for civil servants to engage with research and evidence in some policy fields (health) than in others (justice) and in some countries (UK) than in others. Yet as discussed above, power and contestation remain highly relevant in the framing and problematisation of health issues, with important implications for evidence use. Second, institutions play a role in providing the venues in which such contestation and debate can take place. Institutional arrangements thus provide opportunities in terms of policy spaces where actors with access to these spaces can engage in issue construction and contestation processes. These processes may see stakeholders actively utilising pieces of evidence to problematize issues, but the resultant constructions will also establish frames of understanding that will have further implications for how different pieces of evidence are judged relevant to policy debates. For example, contestation of e-cigarette policy that in England largely played out within the scientific community and government public health bodies, in Germany led to legal challenge, so that the court system became the principal arena for contestation. This consequently limited the policy options for e-cigarette regulation in Germany, with little acknowledgement of the limited knowledge and research available at the time on the effects of e-cigarettes.

Third, while providing arenas for contestation and issue construction, institutional arrangements also serve to establish limits, with only certain actors having access to these spaces, or with the strength of norms and rules providing boundaries on how policy actors might shape and frame evidence to inform policy decisions. For example, Chap. 9 explored the roles of the judiciary and legislature and how these can play important roles in health policymaking and thus evidence use. As would be expected, those institutional arrangements regularly see contestation and debate, but they also shape and limit which types of actors and which types of arguments are made in relation to evidence use.

Reframing Evidence Based Policy Making for the Public Health Sector

Health sector actors regularly speak of the need to use evidence to achieve their goal of improving individual and population health. However, as has been discussed, what evidence use actually means can take a variety of forms and means different things in different contexts. Thus there is a need for more explicit reflection on what sorts of evidence use might best serve health sector goals, as well as recognition of the ways that public health actors' conceptualisations of evidence use may be insufficient given the realities of the policy process.

The health sciences are in many ways deterministic, in as much as clinical medicine and epidemiology build on investigations of the natural world and physical bodies, and often seek to identify direct cause-effect relationships affecting human morbidity and mortality. Many key actors in the health sector have thus been trained in disciplines that look to control for context when considering interventions in order to be able to say 'what works' to reduce illness and improve health. From this perspective, it may seem logical or self-evident that strategies to increase evidence use will translate into more effective policies and interventions. Yet this fails to appreciate the existence of multiple relevant bodies of evidence and multiple ways in which that evidence may feed into complex policy decisions, in which health policy debates cannot be separated from the wider political context.

The fact that evidence use has many meanings is not a new insight, of course. However, this volume moves beyond a mapping of possible uses, to explore how different forms of evidence and evidence use arise and play out in relation to different issues and in different policy contexts. The case studies presented here illustrate how evidence use is shaped by various aspects of the policy, the institutional context in which policy decision are taken and the active agency of policy actors which will seek to frame perceptions of policy problems and their solutions in different ways, which impact in turn on the ways in which different bodies of evidence feed into the policy decisions.

A key message for health policy actors is to take on board the insights from policy analysis presented in this volume and appreciate the contextual nature of evidence informed policy making and the dependence of policy debates on issue and policy framing. This would move debates in this area beyond the identification of politics as a barrier to evidence use, to identify political contestation as a necessary and unavoidable characteristic of the policy process, which provides the context in which evidence use occurs. As we cannot move beyond, or step outside of politics, as some would hope, we must develop a more nuanced understanding of how evidence use occurs in the context of political contestation.

For those concerned with the use of evidence to achieve health improvements, this perspective can help to develop strategies which facilitate forms of evidence use that serve to identify the most efficient and effective solutions to accepted policy problems. It can also, however, serve as a means of facilitating the resolution of protracted policy conflicts. Indeed, a more widespread appreciation of the contested and political nature of policy making, and the existence of multiple framings of policy debates, amongst policy actors could potentially lead to more constructive forms of engagement in areas of vehement political contestation (such as the current debates about e-cigarettes in the UK); rather than seeing opposing sides of debates both selecting pieces of evidence on which to claim an 'evidence based' position (while simultaneously ignoring or dismissing their opponents claims over evidence). Understanding that different accounts of policy evidence result from different assessments of policy concerns and policy framings, may be one way to address the political polarisation over issues and increase the chances that competing actors seek effective policy solutions in good faith.

FUTURE RESEARCH AGENDAS

The current volume identifies a number of potential directions for future research which build on the insights presented here. While the GRIP-health programme, from which this volume emerged, attempted to sample a range of countries with differing levels of economic development and with differing forms of constitutional and institutional arrangements, the scope of analysis and comparison between cases was limited by the time and data available within an ambitious multi-country study. More focussed work should thus be undertaken to explore the different elements of evidence informed policy making that our chapters identify in greater depth, with significant scope for further comparative, politically informed studies of evidence use in low, middle, and high income settings.

For example, while Chap. 10 draws out lessons from aid-recipient settings, there are many further investigations that could be explored along these lines, including to investigate the governance implications of many new donor supported efforts to build systems of evidence use in low-income settings. Even when not reliant on donor support, we are also seeing the development of new domestic administrative arrangements in relation to evidence use occurring in many low and middle income settings. These developments could provide a number of cases to explore how new arrangements governing evidence use are established and embedded and can provide a number of insights around institutionalisation of evidence advisory systems in these settings.

In higher income settings, there is also scope for further comparative work to gain insights into how different national political institutions (e.g. unitary vs federal systems) may interact with the establishment of evidence advisory systems at both national and sub-national levels. Indeed, even though two of our country case studies were federal systems (Germany and Ethiopia) the scope of work covered in this volume was unable to explore systems of evidence use below national levels to any significant degree. There will also be scope to reflect on different types of political systems and the degree to which they allow open contestation surrounding policy issues and whether or how this affects uses of evidence. Indeed, there is a need to go beyond the usual comparisons of countries that are seemingly similar in socio-economic terms and to think across low, middle and high income settings in a globalised world.

Approaches such as these could add much needed insights into how political and institutional factors work to shape the meaning of evidence utilisation in different settings, potentially offering lessons for those actors interested in improving evidence use according to one or another set of normative goals. At present, much public health literature remains focussed on the quality of evidence as judged by technical merits of research design, with broad calls for uptake of high quality evidence often made without consideration of the policy realities involved. As policy actors in the health field increasingly recognise that evidence utilisation is governed by systems working within political environments, they will need insights from work such as this to inform their efforts to improve the governance of evidence systems.

References

Bero, Lisa A. 2005. Tobacco industry manipulation of research. *Public Health Reports* 120 (2): 200–208.

Buchanan, David, Susan Shaw, Amy Ford, and Merrill Singer. 2003. Empirical science meets moral panic: An analysis of the politics of needle exchange. *Journal of Public Health Policy* 24 (3/4): 427–444.

Cairney, Paul. 2016. *The politics of evidence-based policymaking*. London: Palgrave Pivot.

Contandriopoulos, Damien, Marc Lemire, Jean-Louis Denis, and ÉMile Tremblay. 2010. Knowledge exchange processes in organizations and policy arenas: A narrative systematic review of the literature. *Milbank Quarterly* 88 (4): 444–483. https://doi.org/10.1111/j.1468-0009.2010.00608.x.

D'Souza, Bianca, and Justin Parkhurst. 2018. When 'good evidence' is not enough: A case of global malaria policy development. *Global Challenges*. https://doi.org/10.1002/gch2.201700077

Davies, Huw T.O., Sandra M. Nutley, and Peter C. Smith. 2000. *What works? Evidence based policy and practice in public service*. Bristol: Polity Press.

Epstein, Steven. 2006. The new attack on sexuality research: Morality and the politics of knowledge production. *Sexuality Research and Social Policy* 3 (1): 1–12. https://doi.org/10.1525/srsp.2006.3.1.01.

Hammersley, Martyn. 2013. *The myth of research-based policy and practice.* London: Sage.

Hawkins, Benjamin, and Arturo Alvarez Rosete. 2017. Judicialization and health policy in Colombia: The implications for evidence-informed policymaking. *Policy Studies Journal.* https://doi.org/10.1111/psj.12230

Jasanoff, Sheila, and Dorothy Nelkin. 1981. Science, technology, and the limits of judicial competence. *Jurimetrics Journal* 22: 266.

Keane, Helen. 2003. Critiques of harm reduction, morality and the promise of human rights. *International Journal of Drug Policy* 14 (3): 227–232. https://doi.org/10.1016/s0955-3959(02)00151-2.

Khan, Mishal S., Ankita Meghani, Marco Liverani, Imara Roychowdhury, and Justin Parkhurst. 2017. Influences of external donors on national health policy processes: Experiences of local policy actors in Cambodia and Pakistan. *Health Policy and Planning* 33 (2): 215–233.

Lee, Kelley, Anna B. Gilmore, and Jeff Collin. 2004. Looking inside the tobacco industry: Revealing insights from the Guildford Depository. *Addiction* 99 (4): 394–397. https://doi.org/10.1111/j.1360-0443.2004.00718.x.

Lyons, Maryinez. 1999. Medicine and morality: A review of responses to sexually transmitted diseases in Uganda in the twentieth century. In *Histories of sexually transmitted diseases and HIV/AIDS in Sub-Saharan Africa*, ed. Philip W. Setel, Milton Lewis, and Maryinez Lyons. Westport: Greenwood Press.

March, James G., and Johan P. Olsen. 2006. The logic of appropriateness. In *The Oxford handbook of public policy*, ed. Michael Moran, Martin Rein, and Robert E. Goodin, 689–708. Oxford: Oxford University Press.

Marmot, Michael G. 2004. Evidence based policy or policy based evidence? Willingness to take action influences the view of the evidence – Look at alcohol. *British Medical Journal* 328 (17 April): 906–907.

McCambridge, Jim, Benjamin Hawkins, and Chris Holden. 2014. The challenge corporate lobbying poses to reducing society's alcohol problems: Insights from UK evidence on minimum unit pricing. *Addiction (Abingdon, England)* 109 (2): 199–205.

McCormack, Brendan, Joanne Rycroft-Malone, Kara DeCorby, Alison Hutchinson, Tracey Bucknall, Bridie Kent, Alyce Schultz, Erna Snelgrove-Clarke, Cheyl Stetler, Marita Titler, Lars Wallin, and Valerie Wilson. 2013. A realist review of interventions and strategies to promote evidence-informed healthcare: A focus on change agency. *Implementation Science* 8 (1): 107.

McKibben, Heather Elko. 2010. Issue characteristics, issue linkage, and states' choice of bargaining strategies in the European Union. *Journal of European Public Policy* 17 (5): 694–707.

Mitton, Craig, Carol E. Adair, Emily McKenzie, Scott B. Patten, and Brenda W. Perry. 2007. Knowledge transfer and exchange: Review and synthesis of the literature. *The Milbank Quarterly* 85. https://doi.org/10.1111/j.1468-0009.2007.00506.x.
Nutley, Sandra M., Isabel Walter, and Huw T.O. Davies. 2007. *Using evidence: How research can inform public services*. Bristol: The Policy Press.
Nutley, Sandra, Alison Powell, and Huw Davies. 2013. *What counts as good evidence?* London: Alliance for Useful Evidence.
Oliver, Kathryn, Simon Innvaer, Theo Lorenc, Jenny Woodman, and James Thomas. 2014. A systematic review of barriers to and facilitators of the use of evidence by policymakers. *BMC Health Services Research* 14 (1): 2.
Oshitani, Shizuka. 2013. *Global warming policy in Japan and Britain: Interactions between institutions and issue characteristics*. Manchester: Manchester University Press.
Parkhurst, Justin. 2013. The subtle politics of AIDS: Values, bias, and persistent errors in HIV prevention. In *Global HIV/AIDS politics, policy, and activism*, ed. Raymond A. Smith, 113–139. Santa Barbara: Praeger.
Parkhurst, Justin. 2017. *The politics of evidence: From evidence based policy to the good governance of evidence*. Abingdon: Routledge.
Parkhurst, Justin, David Chilongozi, and Eleanor Hutchinson. 2015. Doubt, defiance, and identity: Understanding resistance to male circumcision for HIV prevention in Malawi. *Social Science & Medicine* 135: 15–22.
Rhodes, Tim, Anya Sarang, Peter Vickerman, and Matthew Hickman. 2010. Policy resistance to harm reduction for drug users and potential effect of change. *BMJ* 341. https://doi.org/10.1136/bmj.c3439.
Russell, Jill, Trisha Greenhalgh, Emma Byrne, and Janet McDonnell. 2008. Recognizing rhetoric in health care policy analysis. *Journal of Health Services Research & Policy* 13 (1): 40–46. https://doi.org/10.1258/jhsrp.2007.006029.
Shiffman, Jeremy. 2007. Generating political priority for maternal mortality reduction in 5 developing countries. *American Journal of Public Health* 97 (5): 796–803.
Shiffman, Jeremy, Kathryn Quissell, Hans Peter Schmitz, David L. Pelletier, Stephanie L. Smith, David Berlan, Uwe Gneiting, David Van Slyke, Ines Mergel, and Mariela Rodriguez. 2015. A framework on the emergence and effectiveness of global health networks. *Health Policy and Planning* 31 (suppl_1): i3–i16.
Smith, Katherine. 2013a. *Beyond evidence based policy in public health: The interplay of ideas*. Basingstoks: Palgrave Macmillan.
Smith, Katherine. 2013b. Understanding the influence of evidence in public health policy: What can we learn from the 'tobacco wars'? *Social Policy & Administration* 47 (4): 382–398.

Tong, Elisa K., and Stanton A. Glantz. 2007. Tobacco industry efforts undermining evidence linking secondhand smoke with cardiovascular disease. *Circulation* 116 (16): 1845–1854. https://doi.org/10.1161/circulationaha.107.715888.

Ulucanlar, Selda, Gary J. Fooks, Jenny L. Hatchard, and Anna B. Gilmore. 2014. Representation and misrepresentation of scientific evidence in contemporary tobacco regulation: A review of tobacco industry submissions to the UK government consultation on standardised packaging. *PLoS Medicine* 11 (3): e1001629. https://doi.org/10.1371/journal.pmed.1001629.

Wald, Kenneth D., James W. Button, and Barbara A. Rienzo. 2001. Morality politics vs. political economy: The case of school-based health centers. *Social Science Quarterly* 82 (2): 221–234.

Weiss, Carol H. 1979. The many meanings of research utilization. *Public Administration Review* 39 (5): 426–431.

———. 1982. Policy research in the context of diffuse decision making. *The Journal of Higher Education* 53: 619–639.

———. 1991. Policy research: Data, ideas, or arguments. In *Social sciences and modern states: National experiences and theoretical crossroads*, ed. Peter Wagner, Carol Hirschon Weiss, Björn Wittrock, and Hellmut Wollmann, 307–332. Cambridge: Cambridge University Press.

Open Access This chapter is licensed under the terms of the Creative Commons Attribution 4.0 International License (http://creativecommons.org/licenses/by/4.0/), which permits use, sharing, adaptation, distribution and reproduction in any medium or format, as long as you give appropriate credit to the original author(s) and the source, provide a link to the Creative Commons license and indicate if changes were made.

The images or other third party material in this chapter are included in the chapter's Creative Commons license, unless indicated otherwise in a credit line to the material. If material is not included in the chapter's Creative Commons license and your intended use is not permitted by statutory regulation or exceeds the permitted use, you will need to obtain permission directly from the copyright holder.

INDEX

A
Accountability, 14, 28, 75–88, 92, 116, 172, 186, 188, 189, 192, 196, 203, 204, 224
Adjudication, 113, 114, 121, 125–127, 129, 130
Agenda setting, 129, 140, 210, 228
Agriculture, 13, 41, 52, 55, 59, 61, 62, 66, 210
Aid agencies, vi, 15, 23, 33, 34, 37, 39, 41, 42, 52, 57, 81–83, 87, 88, 163, 166–168, 174, 175, 177–179, 201–216, 224, 225, 229, 230, 234
Aid-dependent, 15, 177, 178, 201–216
Alcohol industries, 8, 228
Arm's length public health bodies, 177

B
Basic Law (*Grundgesetz*), 171
Bounded rationality, 7

Britain, v
Bundesrat, 114, 115, 121, 190
Bundestag, 114, 115, 120, 121, 190
Bureaucracy, 84, 117, 163, 173

C
Cambodia, viii, 13, 15, 21–44, 165–167, 174, 175, 177, 179, 188, 189, 191, 196, 202, 206–210, 212, 213, 229
Cochrane collaboration, 2, 28
Colombia, viii, 13, 14, 91–106, 164–165, 169, 174, 175, 178, 188–191, 193–195, 197, 224, 225, 231
Commissioning research, 170, 176
Committees, 25, 55, 86, 95, 98, 112, 113, 115, 117, 120–125, 163, 170–173, 191–193, 197, 224, 227, 230
Complaint of unconstitutionality, 194

Comprehensive rationality, 7
Conditionality, 202–204, 211, 215
Conflict, v, 4, 8, 54, 61, 66, 67,
    91–93, 116, 119, 124, 140, 141,
    146, 163, 186, 194, 204, 225,
    226, 228, 233
Congress, 36, 93, 95–104, 190,
    191, 193
Constitution, 93–97, 99, 167, 193
Constitutional Court, 96, 97, 178,
    193–195
Constitutional law, 186, 188
Contestation, vii, 5, 8–11, 13–15, 23,
    25, 38, 40, 42, 44, 78, 87, 98,
    105, 130, 146, 223–235
Corporatist system, 112, 116, 130, 178
Corruption, 92
Cost-effectiveness studies, 33
Courts, 92, 96, 97, 103, 114, 117,
    121, 123, 125–127, 129, 130,
    175, 178, 180, 187, 190,
    193–197, 231, 232

D
Department of Health, 170, 192
Development partners, 34, 77, 82,
    162, 163, 166–168, 176, 208
Donor, *see* Aid agencies; Development
    partners
Dual use, 143

E
Electronic cigarettes (e-cigarettes), 14,
    137–147, 226, 232, 234
    policy, 14
Embeddedness, viii, 10, 15, 53, 92,
    103, 106, 112, 117, 139, 159,
    166, 172, 231, 234
England, viii, 10, 13, 117, 138, 140,
    169–170, 172, 174–177, 179,
    187, 189, 190, 194–196, 224,
    226, 232

Enlightenment, 5, 212, 213
    model, 5
Epidemiological modelling,
    33, 40, 209
Epistemic power, 204, 213
Ethiopia, viii, 13, 15, 52–68,
    167–169, 174, 175, 177, 188,
    196, 202, 206, 208, 210,
    212–214, 225, 231, 235
Ethiopian Public Health Institute
    (EPHI), 54, 57, 168
European Union (EU), 57, 59, 66,
    138, 139, 161, 228
Evaluation process, 76, 78
Evidence, vi, 6, 14, 22, 25, 31, 38, 43,
    58, 67, 76, 85, 91, 114, 124,
    141, 160, 165
    advisory systems, 13, 15, 156, 159,
    160, 163, 167, 170, 173, 174,
    178–180, 224, 230, 234
    synthesis, 87, 221
    use of, v, 139
    use within the policy process,
    209–211
Evidence-based advocacy, 204
Evidence-based medicine (EBM), 1–4,
    10, 124, 126, 206, 221
Evidence-based policy (EBP), vi, 1–4,
    7–9, 12, 13, 38, 39, 42, 43, 52,
    76, 88, 111, 112, 115, 130, 139,
    142, 146, 187, 204, 222,
    232–234
Evidence-based policymaking, vi, 7,
    12, 76, 222
Evidence-informed policy, v, vi, 43,
    52, 137–147, 169, 176, 222,
    223, 227, 233, 234
Evidence-informed policymaking, v,
    43, 176, 222
Executive, vi, 78, 92, 95–97, 99–101,
    162, 169, 185, 186, 188,
    190–196
Exercise of power, 206, 213
Experimental studies, 124, 127

INDEX 241

F
Federalist, 187
Federal Joint Committee (GBA), 113–117, 119–130, 171–173, 224, 227
Federation, 167, 187
Frame reflection, 141, 147
Framework Convention on Tobacco Control (FCTC), 24, 30, 32, 38, 39
Framing, 8, 9, 13–15, 22, 26, 30, 39, 42, 43, 51–68, 140–142, 144, 147, 207, 209, 210, 214, 226, 227, 230, 231, 233, 234

G
Gaviria, César, 99, 100, 104, 105
Germany, v, viii, 13, 14, 111–130, 170–174, 176, 178, 179, 188–190, 194, 195, 197, 224, 226, 230–234
Ghana, viii, viii, 13, 15, 75–88, 162–164, 174, 175, 178, 179, 188–190, 192, 196, 202, 206, 207, 211, 213, 214, 224, 229, 230
Ghana Health Services (GHS), 77–82, 84, 85, 162, 163, 213, 214
Governance, 14, 56, 75–88, 92, 130, 156, 157, 160, 164, 165, 170–172, 175, 178, 186–189, 196, 197, 202, 203, 206, 215, 216, 226, 230, 234, 235
  of use of evidence, 11
Governing institutions, 203, 215
Government Midwifery Incentive Scheme (GMIS), 23, 35–37, 206

H
Harm reduction, 141–144, 146, 226, 228
Health Evidence, 34, 155–180
Health policy subsystem, 93, 98–99, 106
Health sector planning, 14, 156, 161, 175, 179, 207
Health Summit, 82–85, 87–88, 211
Health system, 4, 10, 14, 23, 28, 40, 61, 78, 79, 82, 83, 91–107, 156–158, 161, 162, 164–166, 168, 170–173, 176, 185–190, 196–197, 225, 226, 231
  governance, 83, 156, 170–172, 185–190, 196, 197
Health technology appraisal (HTA), 117, 128, 161, 163, 169, 174, 175, 221
Hierarchies of evidence, 2, 22, 38, 231
HIV/AIDS, 2, 13, 23, 24, 27, 32–37, 39, 41–43, 161, 165, 206, 208–210, 229
Holistic assessment tool, 81–85, 87

I
Ideas, vii, viii, 3, 7, 11, 12, 15, 22, 23, 25, 26, 36, 52, 53, 57, 66, 87, 100, 115, 158, 204, 205, 211, 213, 230, 2226
Indicators, 58, 62, 66, 81, 82, 84–86, 88, 92, 119, 124, 168, 204, 207, 210, 211
Influence, vii, 3, 5, 7, 8, 11, 14, 15, 17–179, 186, 189, 191, 201–203, 205–216223
  of donors, 202, 208, 209, 212, 214, 215
Institute for Health Technology Assessment (IETS), 103, 165, 175, 194, 224
Institute for Quality and Efficiency in Health Care (IQWiG), 112, 118, 119, 124, 127, 128, 172

Institute for Quality Assurance and Transparency in Health Care (IQTIG), 172, 176
Institutional analysis, 10, 230–232
Institutional arrangements, 10–13, 15, 23, 53, 130, 158, 174, 177, 178, 224, 230–232, 234
Institutionalist, 42, 91
Institutional logics, 26, 38, 40, 42, 63, 68
Institutional settings, vii, viii, 23
Institutional structures, viii, 11, 12, 24, 52–68, 176, 179, 215, 223, 224
Institutional systems of evidence advise, 158–160
Institutions, 7, 10, 11, 66, 139, 230, 187207
  of the state, 185–199
Instituto de Evaluación de Tecnologíca en Salud (IETS, Institute of Health Technology Assessment), 164–165
Instrumental approaches, 6, 11
Instrumental model, 223
Instrumental use, 6, 12, 115, 189, 224, 226
Instrumental uses of evidence, 223–224
International aid donors, 15
International Development Partners (DP), 77, 166, 176
International donor agencies, vi, 57, 81
International donors, vi, 41, 51, 57, 81–83, 88, 163, 201, 202, 206, 229, 230
Issue construction, 15, 227, 230, 232
Issue framing, 8, 30, 52–68, 140–142, 227, 230

J
Judicialisation/judicializiation, 103, 178, 231
Judiciary, vi, 14, 15, 92, 129, 130, 156, 164, 185–197, 232

K
Knowledge construction, 212
Knowledge-driven model, 5, 212, 223

L
Lancet nutrition series, 59
Law, 31, 32, 35, 92–99, 101–106, 112, 114, 121–127, 130, 171, 172, 186–188, 191, 193–195, 227
Law 100, 98–101, 105, 191
Legislative branch, 96, 97, 178
Legislative framework, 114, 119, 169, 189
Legislature, 12, 14, 15, 86, 91–107, 156, 160, 186, 189, 191, 193, 196, 197, 230, 232
Legitimacy, 76, 77, 87, 88, 93, 96, 111, 114, 117, 129, 130, 142, 204
Litigation, 194
Local Nongovernment Organizations (LNGOs), 77, 86
Logics of appropriateness, 12, 13, 53, 66, 210, 231
Logics of evidence use, 38–41, 53
Londoño, Juan Luis, 100, 101

M
Malnutrition, 52, 55, 58, 59, 62–65, 210, 211
Medical devices, 138–140, 144, 145, 169
Medicines and Healthcare Products Regulatory Agency (MHRA), 139, 169
Minimum service volumes in hospitals, 14
Minimum volumes, 111–130, 190, 194, 227, 231
Ministerial authority, 156, 178

INDEX 243

Ministries of Health, viii, 14, 15, 83, 155–180, 185, 187, 196, 204
Multi-sectoral approach, 55, 210
Multi-sectoral planning, 13, 56, 225, 231

N
Narratives, 7, 11, 12, 40, 41, 67, 147, 235
National Health Service (NHS), 169, 170, 175, 176, 187, 192, 193, 195, 196
National Institute for Health and Care Excellence (NICE), 117, 139, 169, 170, 172, 174, 179, 194, 195, 224
National Institute of Public Health (NIPH), 165–167, 177
National Nutrition Programme (NNP), 53–55, 58–60, 62–64, 66, 67
New institutionalism, 11, 26
NGO, 33–35, 39, 41, 86, 139
Non-communicable diseases (NCDs), 54, 58, 64, 65, 208
Normative power, 210
Norms, vii, 5, 11, 22, 26, 40, 66, 139, 186, 204, 205, 207, 211, 213, 225, 231, 232
Nutrition, 13, 52–68, 168, 207, 208, 210, 211, 225, 231
Nutrition policy, 13, 52–56, 59, 63–68, 207

O
Obesity, 54, 58, 59, 63–65, 210
Overweight, 54, 58, 59, 63–65

P
Parliament, 62, 77, 86, 93, 104, 105, 114, 115, 119, 120, 126, 129, 163, 169, 170, 173, 185–197, 227

Parliamentary Office of Science and Technology, 190
Parliamentary scrutiny, 192
Performance-based financing (PBF), 13, 24, 28–30, 35–37, 206
Performance monitoring, 76
Policy
  communities, 57
  evaluation, 76–78, 83, 85–88
  problem, 7–9, 25, 53, 62, 68, 105, 111, 139, 141, 223, 225, 226, 228, 230, 233
  relevant evidence, generation or creation of, 207–209
  response, 8, 25, 39, 42, 55, 59, 63, 68, 141, 204, 207, 223, 229
Policy-based evidence, 6, 115
Policy-based evidence-making, 6
Policy-relevant research, v
Political contestation, vii, 15, 98, 223, 225–227, 230, 233, 234
Political ideologies, 225
Political institutions, vii, 7, 10, 12, 22, 96, 186, 203, 230, 234
Political model, 5
Political system, vii, 11, 22, 93, 96, 106, 130, 185, 186, 188, 223, 227, 235
Political use, 115
Post-conditionality, 203, 211
Power, vi, vii, 7–10, 25, 26, 31, 40, 42, 61, 77–79, 81–88, 92, 95, 96, 99, 112, 157, 171, 187, 188, 191, 193, 194, 203–206, 210, 212–216, 231
  and influence, 8, 25, 40, 87, 212, 213
  power/knowledge nexus, 205–206
Practices, v–vii, 2, 3, 5, 6, 9–13, 24, 33, 52, 53, 76, 79, 83, 88, 114, 117, 118, 124, 125, 127, 172, 177, 188, 189, 197, 204, 206, 211, 222, 226, 231, 235

Priority setting, 33, 161, 168, 174, 202, 214
Problem solving, 15, 205, 212, 213, 216
Problem-solving model, 5, 223
of research utilisation, 5
Procedural rules, 120, 124, 125
Public health, 1, 23, 28, 29, 33, 37–39, 42, 54, 57, 60, 66, 78, 80, 100, 101, 138–140, 142–147, 157, 160, 161, 165–169, 177, 178, 189, 192, 193, 205, 210, 223–226, 229, 232, 235
Public Health England, 138, 140, 169, 177, 224

Q
Quality of care, 113, 114, 176

R
Rational-linear, 223
Resistance to influence, 214, 215
Resource allocation, vii, 104, 113, 117, 196, 231
Rights, 11, 12, 37, 92, 98, 99, 104, 140, 157, 164, 171, 188, 189, 193–195, 197, 230, 231
Routine data, 123, 161, 168, 169, 175–176, 179, 207, 208, 211, 216
Routinisation, 211
Rule of Law, 92

S
Santos, Juan Manuel, 99, 103–105
Sector-wide planning, 176
Select Committee on Health, 86, 163, 192
Self-administration, 114, 115, 120, 121, 171–173, 178, 188

Smoking, 27, 30, 32, 38, 39, 42, 138, 142–145, 147, 229
Social courts, 114, 121, 125–128, 195
Sovereignty, 202, 203
State, viii, 1, 4, 26, 32, 36, 55, 64, 65, 83, 88, 92–94, 99, 100, 103, 112, 115, 116, 120–123, 125, 126, 139, 156, 157, 160, 165, 169, 171, 172, 174, 185–197, 202, 203, 226
Stewardship of health systems, 83, 155–180, 187
Stewards of health evidence, 158
Strategic use, 12, 14, 115–117, 128, 130, 225–228
Systems and Routines of Evidence Utilisation, 211–212

T
Tobacco, 7, 8, 13, 22–24, 27, 30, 41, 138, 142, 226
control, 7, 13, 22–24, 27, 30–32, 35, 38, 39, 41, 138, 139, 142–144, 206, 209, 226, 229
industry, 30–32, 38, 42, 43, 142, 145, 226
products, 27, 31, 32, 43, 137, 139, 144
Tobacco Products Directive (TPD), 139, 140
Traditional Birth Attendants (TBAs), 29–30
Transnational tobacco corporations (TTCs), 27, 137
Transparency, 76, 116, 125, 172
Tutelas, 102, 103, 194

U
Undernutrition, 54, 56, 58, 59, 61, 64, 65, 68, 210
United Kingdom (UK), 3, 13, 139, 186, 187

United Nations AIDS
  programme (UNAIDS),
  28, 32, 39
Urgency message, 96, 97
US PEPFAR programme, 39

V
Vaping, 143–145
Volume–outcome relationship, 114,
  123–125

W
Weiss, Carol H., 5, 6, 9, 22, 27, 57,
  76, 115, 205, 212, 213, 223,
  226, 229
World Bank, viii, 59, 92, 165, 166,
  179, 202
World Health Organization (WHO),
  vi, 1, 24, 27, 52, 81, 83, 84, 138,
  156–158, 180, 185, 205
World Health Report
  (WHR), 104, 157, 158

The manufacturer's authorised representative in the EU is Springer Nature Customer Service Centre GmbH, Europaplatz 3, 69115 Heidelberg, Germany. If you have any concerns regarding our products, please contact ProductSafety@springernature.com

Printed and bound by CPI Group (UK) Ltd, Croydon, CR0 4YY
23/03/2026
02076672-0011